I0762898

A Terrible
STRENGTH

A Terrible STRENGTH

The Hidden Crisis of the Black Womb & Your Survival Guide to Healing

KEMI M. DOLL, MD, MSCR

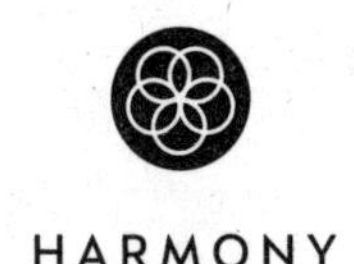

HARMONY

Harmony Books
An imprint of Random House
A division of Penguin Random House LLC
1745 Broadway, New York, NY 10019
harmonybooks.com | randomhousebooks.com
penguinrandomhouse.com

Library of Congress Cataloging-in-Publication Data
Names: Doll, Kemi M. author
Title: A terrible strength / Kemi M. Doll.
Description: New York, NY: Harmony, [2026] |
Includes bibliographical references and index.
Identifiers: LCCN 2025038751 (print) | LCCN 2025038752 (ebook) |
ISBN 9780593977477 hardcover | ISBN 9780593977484 ebook
Subjects: LCSH: African American women—Health and hygiene |
Gynecology—Popular works | Gynecology—Social aspects—United States
Classification: LCC RG121 .D65 2026 (print) | LCC RG121 (ebook)
LC record available at https://lccn.loc.gov/2025038751
LC ebook record available at https://lccn.loc.gov/2025038752

Printed in the United States of America

1st Printing

First Edition

BOOK TEAM: Production editor: Annette Szlachta • Managing editor: Allison Fox •
Production manager: Sarah Feightner • Copy editor: Sara Robb •
Proofreaders: Alicia Hyman, Judy Kiviat, Jill Falzoi, Wes Alspach

Book design by Jo Anne Metsch

The authorized representative in the EU for product safety and compliance is
Penguin Random House Ireland, Morrison Chambers, 32 Nassau Street,
Dublin D02 YH68, Ireland. https://eu-contact.penguin.ie

To all who cramp, bleed, and endure—

and those who love us.

It's time for a new story.

Dear reader,

Welcome in.

What we are going to do here is deep and multifaceted. I have never been a one-note girl and so, like me, this book contains multitudes. I am going to tell you my story—my origins, my traumas (inherited and otherwise), my brainwashing by the medical training system, and how I recovered myself and my womb. It was through this recovery that I found deep respect for the humanity that many wellness practitioners bring to gynecology and womb health. I am an intuitive girl at heart. And yet, this is not an us-versus-them takedown of Western medicine in favor of holistic womb remedies. I love and respect science too much for that. It is science, after all, that I have used, along with my own two hands in surgery, to cure women of womb cancers and save matriarchs of families from departing us too soon. It is science that I have used to administer treatments that finally relieve decades of suffering for women who have been neglected as a societal norm. What you'll find in these pages is a clear critique of the harms of everyday gynecologic care right alongside a passionate defense of the beautiful biology, physiology, and medical discoveries that each and every person with a uterus should know about and benefit from.

Black women's bodies were the soil where so many gynecologic discoveries originated, yet we benefit the least from them. Sometimes I feel we Black women have divested from every type of suffering this society has heaped on us, except that of the womb. Not anymore. I call us to a deeper, more serious examination of our wombs than you'll find in any social media post (including my own). Trends that increasingly resemble popularity cliques, utilizing the marketing style of miracle solutions, are not the answer—not for us. As Black women, we know the truth is much deeper. Black women are unique in our ability to knit friendship and sisterhood so tightly that our bonds are envied by others. With this book, I call us to read, learn, laugh, and cry together to form a new sisterhood—a Womb Sisterhood.

For every person with a womb, this book is vital. We've entered a new era of women's health where we must all be advocates on behalf of our wombs. We know from the powerful work of our social movement leaders that we cannot do any degree of activism alone. So, we won't do this alone either. We are under a relentless onslaught to roll back women's and trans rights, healthcare access, and the dignity we each have to live full and healthy lives. The primary tool of this onslaught is fear. And fear will make you lose the plot. I see it happening already.

When our institutions are crumbling, all we want is certainty. But I'm here to tell you that we won't find it by rejecting science. And to my science purists, we won't help anyone by degrading alternative medicine (or anything that is not in peer-reviewed journals). If you find yourself confused and dismayed by why Black women and others are rejecting gynecologic care, then come inside these pages and listen to their stories. Get out of your echo chamber and listen to what is happening to Black women every single day. Then consider what it means when the violent neglect of the womb Black women routinely face spreads like wildfire across the political arena, as it does now.

Yes, we may all need to be activists—patients, gynecologists, and communities—in partnership.

Thus, I conclude this book with a survival guide to help patients and healthcare providers move forward, providing instructions for both. Black women, I need you to know that respectful, helpful gynecologic care exists, and I've written down what it looks like and how to find it. I have to warn you, though, it starts inside of you and moves out from there.

Ultimately, I am on assignment. It is an ancestral one.

Join me.

Kemi

Contents

CHAPTER 1 Introduction 3

Part I How We Begin: Our Origin Stories

CHAPTER 2 ORIGINS: An Inappropriate Inheritance 17

CHAPTER 3 THE BASICS: Anatomy and our Reproductive Lives 43

Part II How We Live: The Four Conditions of the Womb

CHAPTER 4 HEAVY MENSTRUAL BLEEDING: The Suffering Womb 59

CHAPTER 5 ENDOMETRIOSIS: The Painful Womb 91

CHAPTER 6 FIBROIDS: The Neglected Womb 121

CHAPTER 7 ENDOMETRIAL CANCER: The Deadly Womb. 157

Part III How We Heal: Changing the Script

CHAPTER 8 STRENGTH TO HEAL THE BLACK WOMB 187

CHAPTER 9 WHAT DOES GREAT GYNECOLOGIC HEALTH LOOK LIKE? 202

CHAPTER 10 MYTHS, VOCABULARY, AND POWER 226

A Love Letter to Black Women 239

Acknowledgments 243
Appendix A: A Primer on Finding Quality Gynecologic and Gynecologic Oncologic Physicians 247
Appendix B: 83 Potential Causes of Abnormal Female Genital Bleeding 251
Appendix C: Glossary and Gynecologic Subspecialty List 255
References Cited 267
Index 285

A Terrible STRENGTH

CHAPTER 1

INTRODUCTION

As a Black gynecologic oncologist and scientist, every day I live the reality of the Black womb in crisis. Not the womb in the middle of birth, although God knows Black maternal mortality numbers are shameful, but the *nonpregnant,* everyday Black womb. The womb housed in our bodies that all too often lies like a ticking time bomb in our lives. We are taught to focus on our wombs' ability to get pregnant (or not) and hone our ability to hide anything that comes out of it, except a baby. Meanwhile, the complex ways that the womb functions and can be in dysfunction are ignored, silenced, suppressed, and normalized. Diseases that take years to develop and become severe are "discovered" abruptly at their most destructive, leaving us with few options and reinforcing to the medical establishment the long-enduring belief that Black bodies are inherently broken. The *tick tick tick* of the signs are ignored until the disease explosion arrives. For many, all we hear back is something that sounds like *thoughts, prayers, and birth control pills.*

Some books gently explain the ins and outs of menstruation to pubescent girls, others aim to be an encyclopedia of gynecologic health for everyone, or can promise the secret solutions to overcoming the tumultuous years of menopause. This book is not any of that. This is a vital book for Black women and those who love them. This is a lifesaving resource that aids us in understanding, navigating, and healing from the four primary conditions affecting the Black womb that devastate Black women today—women like your mother, your sister, your aunt, your cousin, your best friend, your wife, and you.

When I refer to *women* in these pages, it is shorthand to mean cisgender women born with a uterus. Trans women are women, full stop. And their reproductive organs, diseases, and journeys are distinct from those who are born with a uterus. And so trans men, gender-fluid, genderqueer, nonbinary, and all those who fall under the gender-expansive umbrella—and were assigned female at birth (AFAB)—will find relevance in these pages. Thus, you will find me using language including both women and individuals / folks / all those with a uterus. However, my expertise is in cisgender women's health, and that is the lens through which my story, my explanations, and my advice is given.

I want to offer to you that gynecologic suffering, what I'll call *Womb Suffering,* is a purely colonial idea, steeped in racist patriarchy. Like most things originating from here, this toxic normalization of Womb Suffering hurts not just Black women but all women and folks of any gender born with a uterus. We are not broken. And we should not live out the consequences of a broken society in our own bodies. It is an inappropriate inheritance.

With this book, I want to reset the norms of gynecologic health in our lives entirely. I want Black women to stop accepting Womb Suffering, just like we don't accept being followed around a store, suspected of stealing. Both insults come from the same place. Just as we have broken loose from the respectability politics of turning the other cheek when disrespected in public spaces, we must break loose from the internalized acceptance of Womb Suffering as intractable, inevitable, or worse, a badge of honor.

When I began medical school, the Black womb was not apparent to me as a locus of crisis for Black women. To me, the womb was a painful inconvenience in my own life, something I barely talked about with friends, and certainly not with family. I was a smart and driven student with a goal of using education to leave behind my homelife forever. By this time, I had already picked myself back up from my rock bottom and had no patience for anything that might make me vulnerable again. I had hardly dated anyone and wasn't having the kind of sex that could get me pregnant. My womb was something that cramped and bled, and that was it. It wasn't until my residency that I began to connect a series of devastating dots around sickness and silence. Dots like learning about the threshold for profound clinical anemia and then seeing Black women at levels far below that who were routinely working full-time with barely livable oxygen levels in their blood. Dots like how common it was for the Emergency Department doctor to suspect pelvic inflammatory disease (PID) caused by sexually transmitted infections, instead of endometriosis, in Black women who dared to show up for help with excruciating pelvic pain. Dots like Black women who'd been seeing their doctors faithfully and routinely for years suddenly diagnosed with stage IV uterine cancer because no one ever asked them about vaginal bleeding.

My OB-GYN residency training was in Chicago, Illinois, at the brand-new Prentice Women's Hospital on the Magnificent Mile, where the labor and delivery rooms were bigger than some city apartments and every floor looked like it was designated VIP. It was in this beautiful environment, where the only thing delineating one patient from another was their race, that I began to see how blatant anti–Black woman medical racism is. Despite all the patients being in nice rooms, I saw the disparity in treatment: Who got drug tested? Whose pain was believed? Who was "high-maintenance" versus "angry and noncompliant"? Who *died*? My colleagues had purposely chosen women's health just like I had, yet the care being offered to all women was not equal. For as much as White women's pain was doubted, Black women's pain was all too often outright denied. For as much as we knew too little about White women's bodies from lack of research, we knew even less about how to treat Black bodies like mine.

This noticing began to add up. At the beginning of my second year of residency, my training program merged with and took over the residency training program at Cook County Hospital, now known as John H. Stroger, Jr. Hospital of Cook County. I split my time between bright and shiny Prentice and older, shabbier Stroger—two hospitals a few miles apart that might as well have been on different planets. It was at Stroger that I first noticed how many Black women were diagnosed with advanced-stage uterine cancer—a cancer that grows in the heart of the womb. This observation led to my first published research project, a simple study comparing the stage of uterine cancer at diagnosis among women at Stroger (majority Black) compared to the National Cancer Database (majority White). There was a striking and fatal disparity: We had many fewer stage I diagnoses and double the number of stage IV cases. Black women were routinely showing up with cancers that spread beyond the womb, where treatment was tough and cures were remote.*

I had chosen OB-GYN to become a surgeon in service of women's health. I wanted to use my expertise to mediate the relationship between a woman and her womb. And yet the more independence I gained in diagnosing and treating the conditions that arise from the uterus, the more I could see, day by day, that there was shocking violence in this most sacred part of the body: hemorrhage, inflammation, fibroids, and cancers. This violence struck Black women the hardest, yet gynecology cared very little about our fate. In medical school, we learned precious little about gynecologic health, much less the specifics of Black women's challenges within it. I am ashamed at the aggressiveness with which I learned in residency to push hysterectomy as the best treatment choice without empathy for the neglectful care that led to years of unnecessary Womb Suffering. How physically draining and humiliating is it to have people constantly think you are pregnant because you are carrying around bowling-ball-size fibroids? What is more vulnerable than sitting in a waiting room, bleeding through your clothes? Black women always had the biggest fibroids, the worst anemia from blood loss, and the most ag-

* In case you look it up, please excuse the vague and pejorative euphemisms for *Black* throughout my very first research paper. I was just beginning to unlearn the racist rhetoric fed to us throughout medical training that suggests that research focused explicitly on Black health equity was somehow less than. I have improved.

gressive cancers. On the days we physicians would explicitly discuss this alarming fact, the answers my teachers gave to my burning questions were no answers at all. "*Black women just don't do well with this,*" followed by, "*We don't really know why.*"

After completing my OB-GYN residency, I knew I needed more tools to deliver the kind of care I desired, so I added more years of training and moved to North Carolina to pursue gynecologic oncology, the subspecialty dedicated to the medical and surgical care of people with cancers of the female reproductive organs. On top of that, I enrolled in a master's program in the UNC Gillings School of Global Public Health—the top program in the country at the time—so I could learn to use the scientific method to identify, dismantle, and rebuild gynecologic care delivery. I wanted every person to experience the highest quality of gynecologic cancer care.

My master's thesis was a study of the role that insurance plays in gynecologic cancer mortality in North Carolina. We sliced and diced the data in many ways to demonstrate how insurance was associated with survival across the different cancers. First, insurance type and quality mattered. At that time, women with private insurance, largely Blue Cross Blue Shield and/or Medicare coverage, had better survival from ovarian, cervical, uterine, and vulvar/vaginal cancers than women with Medicaid insurance. This is a terrible injustice that I fear has only gotten worse, with increased cost and complexity of cancer therapy. Then, when I asked for race-stratified data, I was presented with a graph that I can never unsee. As opposed to all the other cancers, where having private insurance or Medicare was associated with better rates of survival whether you were Black or White, for uterine cancer, it made no difference. Black women, whether they had private, Medicare, or Medicaid insurance, died more than everyone else. By a lot. As I stared at the yawning gap between the lines representing the excess deaths of Black women, year after year and decade after decade, the voices echoed in my head:

"*Black women just don't do well with this.*"

"*We don't really know why.*"

Gynecologic care inequity is not unique to Black women, but is most pronounced for Black women. Like so many other social ills,

Black women, living at the intersection of race and gender oppression, exhibit this reality most clearly. But Latina women experience gynecologic care disparities as do Native American women, and some groups of Asian and Pacific Islander women. Black women are also not a monolith. Black American women who are descendants of United States enslaved peoples have a higher rate of aggressive endometrial cancer compared to Black Caribbean women in their home countries and those who have immigrated to the United States. In geographic areas of deep poverty and social vulnerability, we see worse gynecologic disease and worse gynecologic cancer outcomes for all those who live there. And the specific outcomes of our Black gender-expansive community—those who are nonbinary, trans men, genderqueer, agender, and beyond—are largely left unrecorded in our research where only very recently did sex at birth and current gender identity begin to be collected separately. The "we don't really know why" answer applies to a lot of these groups. And yet I challenge it—because, at some level, we *do* know why. My knowledge comes *from* my scientific expertise on Black women's gynecologic health in this country and comes *through* my lens of being a cisgender Black woman born in the United States.

We are not new to Black women being treated poorly. Serena Williams, arguably the greatest athlete alive in her prime, almost died after giving birth because the nurses caring for her didn't believe her when she said something was wrong with her breathing. She ultimately had a pulmonary embolus that is often fatal if not treated immediately. Beyoncé Giselle Knowles-Carter, arguably the greatest entertainer alive, struggled with preeclampsia and had to undergo an emergency C-section that required months of painful healing and physical therapy to recover from. We are more familiar, now, with the tragic pregnancy stories of Black women, known and unknown before their demise. This is important, but simply woefully incomplete. Black women's wombs are in crisis, especially when we are *not* pregnant. These maternal health stories are the tip of the womb health iceberg. The true magnitude of the toll of gynecologic (nonpregnant) suffering and death that Black women experience in the United States is difficult to fully absorb.

When Jessica Pettway, a young and beautiful social media influencer, died of cervical cancer in 2024, her story went viral. For once, I saw the public dialogue pierced by a story of our nonpregnant gynecologic suffering. Jessica suffered abnormal bleeding and pain for months, with a misdiagnosis of fibroids and, unforgivably, severe delays in receiving a complete pelvic exam to diagnose her advancing cervical cancer. She ultimately died after choosing not to undergo guideline-recommended treatments. She died of a cancer we can nearly completely prevent and cure. This must change.

Ten years into my medical training, I had a breakthrough. At least 80 percent of the Black women I saw suffered from one or more of four conditions: heavy menstrual bleeding, endometriosis (when uterine-like tissue grows outside the womb), fibroids (smooth muscle tumors in the womb), and endometrial cancer (a cancer that grows in the womb). And these four conditions were routinely ignored, missed, or inadequately diagnosed and treated. My awakening of just how much more there was to womb health and how often Womb Suffering was the norm would shape my career and turn me into a world leader in the advocacy for Black women and our wombs.

The Black women I saw in my practice who presented with large fibroids, with heavy bleeding and anemia, and, too often, with endometrial cancer—were coming to me much later than they should have. They were incredibly strong in what they endured, with a terrible ethos of strength before wellness, but that very power was killing them.

Suffering in silence is the normal, default experience of Black women when it comes to our wombs. We see women like our mothers, sisters, and friends suffering in silence and are conditioned to see this as resilience or part of being who we are, instead of a terrible generational inheritance we have yet to break. And the medical establishment does the same. We healthcare providers normalize abnormally heavy periods in young Black women who are up to three times more likely to be walking around with clinical anemia than their White counterparts. And when it comes to extreme pain with periods, Black women are half as likely as White women to get a diagnosis of endometriosis. We normalize debilitating and fertility-destroying fibroids, meaning Black women are up to 80 percent more likely than White women to undergo an early hysterectomy. And when fifty- to seventy-year-old Black women see a few spots of blood long after menopause—a telltale sign of endometrial cancer—they shrug, think, *This is nothing like my twenties,* and keep it moving. They are not worried, and neither are their doctors.

Heavy bleeding, endometriosis, fibroids, or endometrial cancer will affect almost every Black woman we know. The fact is, Black women rarely came to my office with a clarity about their symptoms or their suffering. So, I learned to ask for cues instead. When a twenty-eight-year-old came into the Emergency Department with shortness of breath, heart palpitations, and extremely low blood count (anemia), instead of asking, "Do you have abnormal periods?" [Answer: *No*], I asked, "How many days a month do you *not* bleed?" [Answer: *Six*]. Diagnosis: Severe abnormal uterine bleeding requiring blood transfusions. When a thirty-seven-year-old with an old diagnosis of "asymptomatic fibroids" presented for her routine Pap smear, I noticed what she was wearing. Instead of "Are your fibroids bothering you?" [Answer: *No*], I asked, "How long have you been wearing maternity clothes?" [Answer: *Two years*]. Diagnosis: Large bulky fibroids leaving her at risk for intestinal or bladder compromise. When the sixty- and seventy-year-old women came in, the challenge was greater and the stakes were life or death. Instead of "Any new pain, bleeding, or problems down there?" [Answer: *No, I'm healthy* or *No, I'm clean*], I would say, "Sometimes older women notice they get their periods coming back, or they have new spotting that can pop up. That ever happened to you?" [Answer: *Yes! What is that? I keep some panty liners in my purse just in case.*] Diagnosis: Suspected endometrial cancer.

Our wombs tell the story of how we are weathered by this culture. They tell the story of how we live and how we die. The womb does not just give us life, it can also take our lives. Changing our awareness and response to these four conditions will dramatically impact the health of all Black women and those born with a womb.

This book is a wake-up call, a call to action, and a program for change all rolled into one. My goal is to give voice to the gynecologic distress we have for too long considered normal for Black women and provide us all a survival guide to reset the standard of gynecologic care. Making this shift means becoming freer and stepping fully into the lives we deserve to live, together.

Here is the truth: Most of the information we can find online is geared toward women who have had normal gynecologic health their entire lives. This book is for the rest of us. Sadly, some will take my intentional focus on Black women in these pages to mean this book is not for them. That could not be further from the truth. What we know from all arenas of our society, including civil rights, reproductive health, community organizing, and political power, is that a focus on Black women helps everyone. When we meticulously detail the challenges of racism, sexism, and other forms of oppression that Black women face, we chart a way forward that will benefit everyone. The foundations of gynecologic knowledge in the United States started in the Black body. It's time our reckoning and reclamation of gynecologic well-being center the Black body.

I sit in a few places of tension here, striving to balance how the information and the stories are presented. In being determined to challenge every aspect of normalized Womb Suffering that I see, I worry about being too alarming and creating more fear among Black women who already have enough to deal with. Unfortunately, this hypervigilance is often secondary to our hypervulnerability. There is a reason why 92 percent of Black women voted against the forty-seventh US president when 92 percent of Black women don't agree on any other single thing on the planet. We saw all aspects of the threat, and we knew what was at stake. Whether or not that is a toxic hypervigilance, I am not sure, but I want us to bring that same energy to gynecologic health. This book is to make you aware, so you can make smart moves and do your best for your health.

Another place of tension I feel is in the evidence-based science and the ancestral, spiritual, and emotional knowledge the womb can hold. I love this tension. I pray to God and Jesus is my friend, I set intentions with the new moon,* I firmly believe my massage therapist is a secret Reiki healer, and I beg people to realize that the "natural therapies" versus "toxic medicines" narrative is a scam. The doctor in me says to stick to the evidence. The Black woman in me says the evidence was built in a biased, racist, patriarchal, and violent house. So, I don't try to resolve this tension in these pages, because I don't believe these perspectives must be at odds. I simply strive to be honest. I share data and statistics, alongside stories. I highlight research I think is most relevant to Black women and understanding how we got here—like the link between anger suppression and fibroids, vitamins and endometriosis, and sugar intake and heavy bleeding. I share my thoughts and feelings about medical treatments, including debunking common myths and misunderstandings that keep effective treatments from reaching those who need them most. Some paragraphs give me anxiety when I picture one of my board-certified colleagues reading them. There are sections that I fear may alienate the wellness practitioners who have arisen in the profound gaps that Western medicine has left. I will sit in this tension and hope you all sit with me, and learn. I will tell you where I disagree with a "natural/alternative" trend and where I disagree with my own professional community's guidelines.

My goal, always, is to give Black women tools to unlearn Womb Suffering and the maladaptive behaviors that shorten our lives, and therefore help everyone in the process. Too often, we ignore the signs our bodies give us, and when we do attend to them, we lack the scientific language to name our condition. This book names the biological mechanisms of the nonpregnant womb—how it works and how it goes awry. For both Black women and the medical professionals who care for us, this book will lay bare how the accumulation of racist narratives about our bodies, coupled with our conditioned, collective neglect of our well-being, has created a status quo of gynecologic suffering throughout our lifespans.

Consider this book your invitation to recenter everyday gynecologic health as part of a well-lived life. This is the book I wanted to

* Libra sun, Sagittarius moon, and Libra rising.

give to each of my patients and the book I want every Black woman and person with a uterus to read. It is the book I wish I had when I became fascinated with the womb as a young medical student. In continuing this book, you will understand how we got to a place where Black Womb Suffering is deemed normal (part 1, "How We Begin"), take four harrowing journeys with me and brave Black women who lived the realities of our Terrible Strength (part 2, "How We Live"), and learn the survival guide for how you can recenter womb care, build beautiful bonds of Womb Sisterhood, and never be intimidated by gynecologic science, medicine, or treatments again (part 3, "How We Heal").

Part I

HOW WE BEGIN

Our Origin Stories

CHAPTER 2

ORIGINS

An Inappropriate Inheritance

MY ORIGIN STORY

I am the only granddaughter of Omotayo Olugbemi, who died giving birth. Her name, Omotayo, signifies a child who brings joy to the world. At just three years old, my mother—Omotayo's only surviving child—suffered the trauma of her mother's and never-to-be sibling's death. My grandfather and his subsequent wife never spoke about the loss. My mother faced this yawning chasm of pain and suffering in the silence that surrounded it. She grew up, and then herself almost died after losing a birth. But she survived. And so did I. My grandmother would not live to see joy brought to the world. I am determined to do so.

I've always felt like my identity was a patchwork of *but/and* statements. I was born in Nashville, Tennessee, at Meharry Hubbard Hospital, which was affiliated with one of the few Historically Black College and University (HBCU) medical schools in the country. So, I'm a Black girl from the American South born in one of the Blackest hospitals in the state. But my parents are immigrants from Nigeria. They took advantage of a temporary immigration policy that prioritized admitting educated professionals from African countries to the

United States and avoided what would have otherwise been a harrowing entry to this country. They are Yoruba, and thus, so am I. Yorubas are a tribe known for excess and pride and excellence. Like many of their generation, my parents didn't teach my three siblings and me their language. Perhaps less like others in their generation, my parents' toxicity kept me from forming deep connection with the other Nigerian families in our orbit. We had too many secrets to keep.

When they immigrated, my father was a physician and my mother a nurse midwife. On the surface, I'm the child of highly educated Nigerian immigrants, but peel back one layer and things get complicated. Beneath my father's professional facade lay a far more complicated truth—his life was marked by deception and criminality. He attended medical school in Nigeria and graduated, but that doesn't tell the full story. Starting before I was born and continuing in my childhood, my family members' lives were embroiled in my father's failed scams, one after the other. We moved from city to city every few years, running to escape the consequences of his poorly spun schemes. Eventually, he would end up serving time in jail, finally caught in his web of lies.

My family was not poor. We always lived in big-enough houses, but sometimes they felt empty inside, or we slept on mattresses on the floor. We always had dinner, but at times, all my siblings and I had to share was a box of Bagel Bites, a can of biscuits, and crackers with cheese divided among the four of us. We had running water, even if we didn't always have heat. To this day, I will not take a cold shower—ever. The cold water transports me back to shivering through my daily bathing ritual as a child, asking when we could turn the heat back on, and being told, "When your father gets back." It wasn't about not having the money to pay our bills. My father controlled the family finances with an iron fist, and we couldn't trust him to be responsible.

We also lived in terror. Depending on his mood, my father would either ignore us, eagerly engage us in something he was excited about—usually some news item—or berate us while pitting us against one another. He called us *stupid, selfish,* and *useless,* and often told us we were "not as good as your brother or sister." Sometimes I hear first-generation and immigrant Nigerian millennials joking that insults are a love language in Nigeria. I wish I could laugh along with them, but insults were delivered with pure anger and venom in my home. Each person had their place in the family hierarchy, and points were awarded by punching down. My father's surveillance was constant. He tapped the phone lines and recorded our calls, only to play back particularly embarrassing snippets in cringeworthy "family meetings" while my mother sat by him in silence. My mother survived his manipulative control by bobbing and weaving, telling half-truths to ease his questioning, and teaching us to do the same. Perhaps, these were the lessons she had learned in her own life as a child whose caretakers dared not speak of her mother's untimely death. Speaking of what is wrong or what hurt was simply not done. Her mantra was, "We have to keep the peace." *Peace* was defined by the absence of shouting. *Keeping the peace* meant making my father happy and making him feel justified in his actions, no matter how egregious they were. If he claimed the sky was green, our role was to respond, "Yes, very green, Daddy."

I am aware that I am rupturing the powerful tradition of the silence that is kept around one's homelife and struggles in Nigerian culture. In a way that is even more terrifying to me, I am about to go on and daringly show how I simply did not receive what I needed as a child from my mother. My intention is not disrespect or revisionist history—it is simply to tell my truth and demonstrate how powerful individual moments are in the life of a bright Black girl destined to be a smart Black woman navigating this perilous society.

~

At a very young age, I understood the box into which my family and my culture placed women, and I rejected it entirely. I had three brothers, so my mother and I were the only females in the house. I saw how she worked long overnight shifts as a nursing leader, then came home to cower before my father, work silently in the kitchen, and mute herself when he spoke abject lies. She was my first role model of what a girl grows up to be, but when she looked to me to join her in this small, silenced life, I recoiled. I wanted to reject anything soft, anything kind, and anything that was exclusively for women, even when it appealed to me. It was a constant internal tug-of-war. I was not interested in getting trapped by the boys and men in my life, so I never wanted to be too much of a girl. I believe my mother felt this and received it as a rejection of herself. She told me that I "raised myself" because, as she remembers, I made it clear that I didn't need her. She told me she asked God to send her a girl and he sent her me instead.

Is this why when I told her at twelve years old that my first menstrual cycle lasted nine days and hurt, her face screwed up with confusion and disgust? I remember that day clearly. I had learned about periods a few years earlier from a sex education class organized by my Girl Scout troop leader. In retrospect, this leader was a fairly radical Buddhist White woman subverting much of our oppressive suburban culture in the Deep South. I had learned what naked adult bodies looked like by watching R-rated movies and worse with my older brothers during long stretches where we would be left home alone to fend for ourselves. I saw my first rape scene in a movie in elementary school.* I had nightmares for weeks. My parents did not have a concept of appropriate or inappropriate viewing for children, as was true of many parents in the late eighties and early nineties.

By the time my first period came, I did not consider asking for help from my mother or anyone else. I was already a traumatized hyper-independent child who had learned that showing any vulnerability was an invitation for attack. At home, I was always prepared for a verbal lashing inspired by the most innocent of moments. And middle school was a social hellscape. I was teased mercilessly by my classmates. I had an ever-changing "best friend" who I connected with and shared a sense of being an outsider with—until the time came when they had to choose between being my friend and gaining a modicum of social status. It was also hard because I, like many other girls, had my monthly, secret routine to manage.

* Though I am not sure, through a disturbing Google search of rape scenes in movies in the 1980s, I believe the movie was *The Accused*. This film was based on a true story, won Jodie Foster her first Oscar, and left indelible scars on me.

By eighth grade, my periods were horribly painful. My sharpest memories were the bus rides home from school, sitting in the very first seat because by the end of the day, I could not walk an extra step more than I had to. I would partially recline in that seat, breathing as slowly as possible and wincing with every bump and sway of the school bus. I would stumble off the bus and into our driveway, my shoulders drooping with a heavy backpack full of books, willing myself to climb the stairs and then falling into my bed, at last. I ate ibuprofen like candy and it tore up my stomach for days, but the pain relief was worth it. It happened every month, and the pain never lessened. I just got better at living through it. I didn't realize it at the time, but I was developing the kind of silent resilience that we as Black women are conditioned to endure. The training started early.

I was seventeen when my mom took me to my first gynecology appointment. Nothing prompted it. I think she may have asked whether I thought I should go to a gynecologist and I said yes, because I didn't know why I shouldn't. Was she trying to figure out if I was sexually active? (I wasn't.) It seemed a part of routine healthcare to me, a box to check. We went to the office, and when my name was called, I went back to the exam room by myself. I had no idea what to expect, so I relied on my tried-and-true approaches to navigating an unknown environment—stay quiet, feign nonchalance, and be on guard. I was left to fill out the intake questionnaire, and nothing seemed relevant to my life. *Do you get periods regularly?* Yes. *Do you have any problems with your cycle?* No. *Have you ever had an STD?* No. *Are you trying to get pregnant?* No. The medical assistant asked if I wanted to meet the doctor before my exam. The only exams I had experienced were general physicals from family doctors where they may peek into your underwear to confirm normal genital development, but that was it. Why would I need to see the doctor before she came in to do what doctors do? Was this question a test? "No, it's not a big deal," I said and shrugged. She looked miffed and directed me to get completely undressed, put on a paper sheet, and wait on the table. These instructions took me by surprise, but I wasn't going to show that. I got undressed and waited.

The ob-gyn entered. She was a White, blond, middle-aged woman in a bright pink tweed suit. I did a double take, as she fit no image of a doctor I had in my mind. She offered a tight smile and asked brusquely if I had any questions or concerns. "No." She told me to lie back and inserted the speculum without preamble, took a Pap smear, then did a bimanual exam, inserting one hand inside my vagina with the other pushing on my pelvis. The stretching hurt, the pressure was wholly unfamiliar to me, and the scraping of my cervix was a bright, new pain. I was alone. I stayed still and quiet, following the directions. Hyperaware. She finished, told me to get dressed, and left. As I walked back to the chair where I'd left my clothes carefully folded, I wondered if I was allowed to wipe the jelly lubricant off between my legs, and if so, what was I supposed to use?

I dressed and the nurse came back to lead me to the doctor's consultation office, a dark wood-paneled room. She sat behind a large desk with one of those old-school green-and-gold lamps. I felt like I was in the principal's office. She opened my chart and started talking at the same time. "So, your exam was normal . . ." and trailed off. "Oh," she said, pausing and looking up at me—truly looking at me—for the first time. "This was your first exam?" I nodded. "Oh. Sorry. Well. Everything was fine." She then backtracked to begin describing to me what had happened in the exam room, a typical pelvic exam. What she didn't say, and what I know now as a double board-certified ob-gyn and gynecologic oncologist, is that I had zero indications for an internal pelvic exam. I was not sexually active. I was not of age to have or need a Pap smear. I had reported no problems with my cycle and no gynecologic symptoms. I had never been sexually active and reported no history of sexual abuse. It was my first contact with a gynecologist, and it should have been a helpful, warm exchange of information to begin my gynecologic health journey. It should have been a time to teach me about my body, cycles, what is normal and what is not. It should have been a chance to screen me for any interpersonal relationship abuse and assess my interest and preparedness for future sexual activity. When the ob-gyn and her medical assistant looked at me, I don't know what they saw, but it wasn't anything that inspired care, tenderness, or even curiosity. I was a young Black girl who wasn't pregnant or infected. I had no problem for them to solve. I'm not sure they saw me at all.

OUR ORIGIN STORY

To be a Black woman in the United States is to inherit the story and the consequences of the transatlantic slave trade, personally. Between 1526 and 1867, at least 12.5 million predominantly West Africans were sold as property to work in bondage for the rest of their lives and to birth children who would do the same. For generations, Black women and any Black person with female reproductive organs were the engines of reproducing racial capitalism's most valuable resource during slavery in North America: the Black body. The enslaved workforce, including women who were expected to meet the demands of physical labor on top of the work of childbearing, would produce inordinate wealth for the colonies and eventually the United States for over two hundred years. In the nascent days of gynecology, White male physicians were highly concerned with the ability, effectiveness, and potential disease of the Black womb. They were paid handsomely to examine and ensure its reproductive capacity, even serving as experts in court cases where slave owners accused one another of selling "spoiled" goods: a Black woman with a gynecologic disease.

These doctors also saw in enslaved Black women an opportunity to learn gynecologic anatomy and discover new techniques, as it was considered improper to do so on the bodies of White women. As historian and professor Deirdre Cooper Owens quotes Elaine Breslaw in her book *Medical Bondage,* "White doctors were free to perform procedures on black women that would have been socially unacceptable to white women, at the minimum violating the standard of modesty." Black wombs were profitable and valuable to the White ruling class, whether or not they were attached to a living being. Of particular interest to me, and any of my gynecologic oncology colleagues reading this today, is the story of Mary Reynolds. Dr. Cooper Owens recounts Ms. Reynolds was an enslaved Black woman, who in 1850 became the first person on record in the United States to have a hysterectomy for uterine cancer. Her doctor was Paul Eve, a well-regarded surgeon at the Medical College of Georgia who served as president of the American Medical Society. She died of her cancer three months after the surgery, as it was unlikely that the procedure alone could have cured her advanced condition. Her preserved womb was displayed in Dr. Charles Meigs's Philadelphia medical museum, as a relic of medical research. I am an excellently trained gynecologic oncologist and uterine cancer scientist and grew up in the state of Georgia, where this happened. Never once did I learn that the first surgery for uterine cancer was done on a Black body. This is one of many examples of how Black women's bodies, in particular, served as the founding substance from which gynecologic knowledge was gained. There are many more.

Removal of diseased ovaries was pioneered by Dr. Ephraim McDowell, who performed the first recorded removal on a White wife and mother in the frontier community of Danville, Kentucky. Despite the surgery's success, he would proceed to refine the procedure exclusively on enslaved Black women throughout the Southeast, in the same area in which I was born and on the same land on which I grew up. He would be called the "Father of the Ovariotomy," though this procedure is now called *oophorectomy*. The "Father of the Cesarean Section" was Dr. François-Marie Prevost, who developed his techniques exclusively on pregnant enslaved Black women in Louisiana. Dr. J. Marion Sims, the so-called "Father of American Gynecology," spent years in the mid-1800s developing experimental gynecologic surgical techniques on Anarcha, Lucy, Betsey, and other unnamed enslaved Black women in Montgomery, Alabama, about five hundred miles from where I would clinch my decision to apply to medical school, despite finding myself, at nineteen years old, kicked out of college, with no home to return to. The surgeries performed by Dr. Sims were meant to heal complex urogenital fistulas, a condition in which abnormal connections develop between the bladder, uterus, and vagina, causing urine leakage. This condition was often the result of birth trauma and could render a woman ostracized due to the persistent odor, and ill due to repeated pelvic infections. Dr. Sims performed his operations without anesthesia and felt himself to be these women's benefactors for providing them room, board, and addictive drugs. His story, in particular, highlights a lie that pervaded my clinical training, years after I got myself back on track and did succeed in becoming an Ivy League–educated physician. This lie was woven throughout the decades of research on uterine cancer that I now work to dismantle. The lie says that when laying hands on the Black body to ostensibly treat gynecologic conditions, we physicians, by default, are doing so with respect and good intention. As a Black woman who has endured gynecologic care, I know this is not true. As a Black woman who slowly watched and realized how Black bodies were seen differently from White ones over twelve years of medical training, I know this is not true. Though today, this lie can be subtle, and even unconscious to many in gynecology, I highlight Dr. Sims's willingness to be clear about the disgust he felt for his patients' bodies: "If there was anything I hated, it was investigating the organs of the female pelvis," he shared, starkly, in his autobiography.

In recent years, there has been a moral reckoning inside gynecology to come to terms with this foul history and what it means today—namely, the normalized dehumanization of Black women. The statue of Sims that stood in New York's Central Park has been removed, and tributes to Anarcha, Lucy, and Betsey have been erected. But violence and disregard of the Black body run deep like salted trenches across the field of gynecology.

The National Medical Association is a historically Black institution, formed in 1895 at a time when the American Medical Association refused entry to Black doctors entirely. As recently as 2019, this Black professional organization published in its journal a robust defense of Dr. Marion Sims. Even a Black publication felt the need to make a case for the benefits of Sims's surgical experimentation, proof that today, as throughout history, Black women are too often not protected, even by our own. The techniques of these so-called "fathers of gynecology" set the stage for an entire field's approach of disregard and exploitation of the Black womb. Outside of its role as a site of experimentation, the Black womb would be treated only as a threat and a problem. Our profession's biomedical understanding of disease, the structures of our care delivery, and our behavior toward Black women with gynecologic needs all grew out of this toxic soil. I experienced it firsthand in my medical training to become a gynecologist.

My road to being one of the top OB-GYN residency applicants in the country in 2008 was not a given. Several years earlier, I had failed out of the prestigious Duke University Pratt School of Engineering and had to claw my way back to a decent GPA and a competitive medical school application.

Despite graduating at the top of my medical school class, in so many ways in my mind, I was still fighting. Failing out of Duke had been the first serious and real threat to the lifelong plan I had nurtured since I was five years old. My plan was to escape my family circumstances based on my ability to succeed in school and create the life I want. When I got my final grades in the spring semester of my sophomore year—one F, one WF (withdrew early from the class while I was failing it), one D, and one A*—the ground shifted forever beneath my feet. To me, at the time, the worst had happened. Though I was okay with failing myself in social situations, in failing to be the daughter my mother wanted, and in failing to figure out how to be around my father without getting hurt, I was never supposed to fail at school. It was my golden ticket to freedom and the sole refuge of my hopes for my future. When I received the official academic suspension letter, I was kicked out of school, but I also could not go home.

What had happened to me, the straight-A student who had arrived at college two years earlier? The fighting between my parents had reached a fever pitch after years of erosion of my father's better angels. I feared for my mother's safety and had stood up boldly to my father in a family showdown that would haunt me for years. (I would never speak to my father again.) In retaliation, my father refused to

* My "easy" English literature class . . . I know, I know, I didn't get it yet.

pay my family's portion of my school tuition when I started that sophomore year, so I took out emergency loans and added more work-study hours to stay in school. I drove back and forth between Atlanta, Georgia, and Durham, North Carolina, countless times that year to support my mother and be a buffer presence. I'm not sure I ever actually improved anything, but I tried. And failed. I faced expulsion due to poor academic performance, was required to move off campus within a few weeks, lost my student card and my meal plan all because I failed in my one job—to be good at school.

From that crisis, something was born in me. It started out as survival, grew into a ruthless achievement machine, and has now matured into a depth of certainty for which I am proud and grateful. What was born was a thought: *No matter what happens, I will be okay.*

I did not believe that I would be okay because some divine power would come and save me. I had failed out of school, and no one was coming to my rescue. Nor did I believe that "everything will always work out," because my family was most definitely not working out. I would be okay only for one reason—I would always take the next best step. I would look around, choose the least awful of all choices, and move forward. I felt no guarantees about my future, only that you wouldn't catch me standing still, waiting to be saved. I would figure out plan B after plan A had failed, and figure out plan C after plan B crashed and burned, and so on. The keyword here was *I*. I could rely on no one but me, so I had to protect myself—and I wrapped myself in armor. I began to imagine myself in a second skin that was translucent but strong as titanium.

After losing my student status, and tearfully withdrawing from a planned study-abroad experience in Ghana, I got a job working in the dean's office supporting the philanthropy outreach efforts for the summer. I rented a room in a small townhouse from an older White woman who, in retrospect, I realize probably had developmental delay. She was very childlike and had a bird named Birdie. I bought used dorm room furniture from a consignment store, rented a bed from Rent-A-Center, and lugged along my prized possession: the TV/VCR I had won at a Senior Night raffle at my high school graduation. I roamed around campus like I still belonged there, participated in my sorority's activities like I had a working school ID, and disconnected totally from an utterly broken heart.

I don't know what it was like to be around me during this year, as it is mostly a haze of sadness, anger, and deflecting attention away from myself at all costs. My treasured Delta sorors, an incredible cohort of talented, charismatic, high-achieving Black women, were my sanctuary. They were my exoskeleton. I could roam through campus life tucked deep into their ranks, quiet, and able to feel a bit of laughter, love, and lightness, even if it was secondhand. When the fall semester started back up again, I got a job in the biomedical engineering lab of a professor in whose class I had done well before the ground had started to slip out from underneath me. While I was out of school, my only goal was to get back in.

After I successfully reapplied and was granted readmission, my only goal was to graduate on my original timeline in my originally chosen degree. I had eighteen months to do it. I felt pressure to not be another Black student who "could not handle" engineering. I stacked up a course load and schedule to complete all my degree requirements. I became a studying and note-taking machine. When I proved to myself that I could get A grades again, my only goal was to shoot my best shot at medical school. I enrolled in a summer pipeline program for minority medical students at Columbia University, the kind of program that, as I am writing this, is being dismantled across the country in response to racist "anti-DEI," pro-segregationist rhetoric. After taking summer classes to catch up in biochemistry, I spent eight glorious weeks in New York City in a program run by Dr. Hilda Hutcherson, the dean of diversity at Columbia. When I was later admitted to this Ivy League institution, it was because Dr. Hutcherson insisted that they take a chance on me.

My undergraduate GPA was far, *far* below the class average, and my admission test scores were decent but not stellar. After a year and a half of working at the expense of everything else, I was back on the path of my life plan. I did not have confidence, though. I was not incorporating my successes along the way and seeing my own potential. I was too disconnected from myself for that kind of self-awareness and personal growth. Instead, I had resolve. *No matter what happens, I will be okay.* I will look around, choose the least awful of all choices, and move forward.

I graduated from Columbia University's College of Physicians and Surgeons at the top of my class. I knew I would have my pick of OB-GYN residencies, and I knew where the top programs were at the time: Harvard, University of Pennsylvania, Johns Hopkins, and University of California, San Francisco. I scheduled an interview at the Prentice Women's Hospital of Northwestern Medicine in Chicago, Illinois, first, thinking I'd practice for the more competitive interviews that would come later. To my surprise, I loved my interview day. I was impressed with the faculty and residents, the freestanding women's hospital, the suite of operating rooms, and the high volume of gynecologic surgery that took place there. Most important, I appreciated the absence of a segregated floor for VIPs. I'd learned this was a common feature at other hospitals. One thing that had struck me in medical school was that our hospital treated the uninsured and those with public insurance one way and the privately insured another. I was nauseated by the blatant inequity.

When it came time for me to rank my ideal training programs, I didn't rank any of those top programs first. My advisors were dismayed, as they expected me to aim as high as possible in selecting a postgraduate placement. But I wanted a place with no hierarchy. Naively, I thought I'd found that in Prentice.

I soon came to realize that while Prentice did not have a VIP floor, it did have segregated clinics and an invisible filter on care. The resident training physicians had our own outpatient clinic called Prentice Ambulatory Care, or the PAC. Women with private insurance saw our attending physicians for care in a different building.* These same, more-experienced physicians supervised us, but in the PAC, we could start to take some independence in our decision-making and care delivery. I had mixed feelings. I primarily wanted to serve Black and Brown women, and I loved that I could do so at the PAC clinic. At the same time, I knew it was wrong that these

* People with Medicaid were also seen in our attending's clinic to a much smaller and seemingly tightly regulated degree.

women all had trainees for their primary doctors. I don't think this uniformly resulted in worse quality care or interactions for them. I certainly gave them my best, and due to the supervising doctors, they always had at least two physicians reviewing their records to ensure we were offering the best care. But we know that separate is inherently unequal.

When our patients receiving prenatal care at the PAC clinic came to Prentice's beautiful labor and delivery (L&D) unit, they were labeled outright. *PAC* appeared in big letters next to their names on the digital board that tracked where all patients were in their labor process. With thirty-two L&D rooms, this helped us know which patients were "ours"—belonging to the resident team—and which were private patients of our dozens of attending physicians. Labeling, especially when it comes to healthcare, is a breeding ground for stereotype and biased treatment. My fellow residents and I still cared for the privately insured patients, but only to the degree to which our supervisors wanted our involvement. You do not have to be a sociology scholar to imagine that the PAC patients were treated differently. I was a part of this system.

Based on my conditioning, I was not immune to mistaking a PAC patient's stoicism for lack of pain. I suffered under the same delusion that Black women were stronger than their peers. I personally knew that I carried many hurts, physical and emotional, and yet I was always seen as tough and resilient by my superiors. I didn't yet realize this meant that I needed *more* care, not less. I also knew enough history to know that Black women had survived the unthinkable in slavery. It was not conscious, but I now realize I saw the Black and Brown patients as more resilient than others. I noticed pain only through one lens: what it looked like on White women. Under the supervision of my attending, I discharged a Latina woman who had days of flank pain and inflammatory signs in her urine sample because she slept while she was in the hospital. I couldn't imagine a person in so much pain being able to sleep, because I had never seen a White woman do so. She returned with a severe kidney infection that could have been prevented. I was complicit in the system that taught me, in subtle and overt ways, that Black and Brown bodies had to do more to prove their suffering. We simply would not take their word for it. Though I have deep shame when I think back on a few similarly searing clinical interactions, I recognize that I was a product of my medical education.

There were moments of awareness that started to shift things for me. As I moved along in medical training and rose in the ranks, I could spend more time thinking about the patients I encountered and contemplating the interactions we had, instead of keeping my focus on the endless list of tasks handed to an intern at 5:00 A.M. I'd like to think that this time and experience led to me being more aware and nuanced with my Black patients. Maybe, maybe not. What is certain to me was that my personal experience of being a Black woman resident in an overwhelmingly White training program taught me the most about how Black women were seen differently in medicine.

Not long after I began at Prentice, my program director (my boss) recruited me to help support efforts to diversify our training program. We were in the heart of Chicago, yet there had only been four Black residents total over the prior fifteen years, all within the last two years. Was it a blip, or would we truly commit to representing the city we served? My boss wanted to increase the number of racially and ethnically underrepresented residents in the program and asked me to help. I set out to organize what I had seen be effective when I was out on the residency interview trail myself—social mixers where Black and Brown applicants could meet with Black and Brown trainees, and scheduling to ensure minority applicants had at least one interviewer who could identify with their background. When these routine equity recruitment efforts became known to the larger group, I faced severe backlash spearheaded by a White Latina resident. She excoriated me in a public forum for "introducing bias" into our "fair" application process, and other White residents joined in. My program director said nothing in my defense, nor did any of my colleagues who were present. When I asked my boss why he hadn't publicly supported me, choosing silence rather than standing with me, he told me that he thought I had it under control and was defending myself well. He saw me as strong and felt no inclination to intervene on my behalf.* I will never forget that experience for what it taught me about who I was working with and what field I was in. This environment was one that would celebrate Black excellence but not deign to consider Black humanity. It was a place where after you had been harmed, a good White ally would come sit beside you, but they dared not jump into the fray and risk themselves in the moment. Someone said in that meeting, "What is really *that different* about the Black experience *today*?" Someone else said, "What about *White Muslims*? Why don't you care about them?" I did my best to respond with passion and conviction, holding my dignity close and refusing to let loose the angry tears that threatened to fall. Immediately afterward, I sought solace with a phone call to a fellow Black resident who had not been present but could validate my feelings of betrayal. Then, I fixed my face and went on to work my full clinical day back under the limelight of the supervising physicians, back to the routine of performing at my very best, with little margin for error and even less grace. I'm sure I was excellent.

That night, I went home, cried, raged, and went to bed. I woke up the next morning with a different awareness of how my fellow gynecologists-to-be saw Blackness and Black people. They could not see how much the world demands of Black women while simultaneously giving nothing back to us, except the assumption that we can handle it. I could see it, though. I had felt it, violently, and my long journey to fully reclaiming my voice and my body began.†

In 2016, a study of over two hundred University of Virginia medical students and residents indicated that between 22 and 42 per-

* A few colleagues approached me right after the verbal attacks to let me know, privately, that they supported me. All Black women who have worked in predominantly White environments will recognize this cowardly ritual.

† Like most Black people in these United States, I have absolutely zero desire to time travel to the past. But my big, grown, forty-three-year-old self sometimes daydreams about standing next to twenty-six-year-old Kemi and giving the colleagues that were in that room the verbal excoriation I am now quite capable of. Mostly, though, I think about how today, each and every one of them are board-certified ob-gyns, and that day—they won.

cent of them (based on the level of training they'd achieved) believed that Black people had biologically thicker skin than White people. For clarity, these doctors and aspiring doctors believed Black people literally had denser epidermis. (This is false.) The researchers went on to demonstrate that holding false biological beliefs about Black people resulted in less accurate pain assessments and greater racial bias in pain treatment. We see the impact of such ignorance in daily healthcare practices. In a 2019 study of 1,701 postpartum women in a North Carolina hospital, led by Dr. Jasmine Johnson, Dr. Alison Stuebe, and colleagues, Black and Latina women had fewer routine assessments of their pain by their healthcare teams, despite expressing severe pain levels equal to or higher than White women's. These women were also less likely to receive pain medication within the first forty-eight hours after giving birth. In studies of people dying of cancer with intractable pain, Black people still don't receive adequate pain or anti-nausea medications or other supportive care to ease the end of their lives. We are presumed to be strong, to not need the same level of care, tenderness, and love extended to others.

Here is the thing. Black women *are* strong. If we weren't, we wouldn't be here. The unique strength of Black women, passed down generation after generation, has been studied extensively. I'm drawn to the work of Dr. Cheryl Woods Giscombé, an accomplished nurse with a PhD in social and health psychology who has conceptualized what she calls the *Superwoman Schema* among Black women. In her groundbreaking article, she writes, "racism . . . during and after legalized slavery in the United States—forced African American women to take on the roles of mother, nurturer, and breadwinner out of economic and social necessity." She later continues, "The legacy of strength in the face of stress among African American women might have something to do with the current health disparities that [we] face." Dr. Giscombé's work recognized that this superwoman strength has emotional, psychological, and physical implications. Pulling from the scholarship of Black feminist thought since the 1970s, she formalized the Superwoman Schema to help us think about the impact of Black women's strength on our health.

The superwoman's burden has five components: 1) an obligation to manifest strength; 2) an obligation to suppress emotions; 3) resistance to being vulnerable or dependent; 4) determination to succeed despite limited resources; and 5) an obligation to help others. Black women adopt these ways of being in response to the historical legacy of racial and gender stereotypes and oppression, past personal mistreatment or abuse, and lessons received from our foremothers. In research studies, women who score high on Superwoman Schema scales have poorer sleep, higher blood pressure, and signs of premature cellular aging. Black women report postponing their self-care in service of other obligations, while knowing the related stress is impacting their health. Our migraines, hair loss, panic attacks, weight gain, diabetes, depression, and other chronic health conditions all make manifest the overwhelm that we're carrying. And we are celebrated for it.

My contribution to the scholarship produced by Dr. Giscombé and others is to shine a light directly on the relationship between the Superwoman Schema and gynecology. Others have made the connection to pregnancy complications, but rarely to gynecology. I have observed that younger generations have started to push back against or reject the superwoman identity in many parts of their lives. I see Black women online divesting from the expectation of putting everyone's needs before their own. Paying attention, especially to mental health and well-being, is now normalized in Black women's gatherings. I am inspired by the work of Nedra Glover Tawwab, author of *Set Boundaries, Find Peace,* and Dr. Joy Harden Bradford, founder of Therapy for Black Girls. I applaud this progress. But I fear without the clear understanding of how this superwoman identity also shows up in our gynecologic health, we may continue to resist vulnerability in this arena even as we make strides elsewhere.

And we must not forget the Black church, a central influence on Black culture, whether one personally ascribes to Christian teachings or not. The standard of the good, churchgoing Black woman who did life in the "right" order (husband, kids, then joy) leaves no space to explore gynecologic well-being beyond pregnancy control. In many ways, the Black church culture is a robust defense against the legacy of hyper-sexualization of Black women by White society. But it is often a defense levied by silencing and shame of *any* sexuality for Black women at all. And when common treatments for debilitating gynecologic conditions are so often and frustratingly lumped together as "birth control"—the treatments for Womb Suffering take on a stigma unto themselves and become psychologically beyond the reach of so many good church girls who are suffering.

Across nearly every single major womb condition, Black women are more likely to have severe disease, less likely to respond to treatment, and, in the case of womb cancers, much more likely to die. After covering our origins in this chapter and the basics of reproductive anatomy and function in chapter 3, we will embark on a storytelling journey to see this up close and personal. In part 2 of this book, we will take a deep dive into four key gynecologic conditions affecting Black women: heavy menstrual bleeding, endometriosis, fibroids, and uterine (endometrial) cancer. For each condition, I will show that we often miss the signs and override our bodies' cries for help in part because our foremothers taught us a self-sufficiency that can keep us from demanding adequate attention and care. Our families praise our matriarchs for being strong yet are silent about what killed them. I learned strength as self-sufficiency in my own childhood home and perhaps as my own mother had learned the same in hers. In a world where no one cares about your womb, self-sufficiency means normalized Womb Suffering.

ORIGINS OF THE GYNECOLOGIC HEALTHCARE SYSTEM

The medical community understands human biology and disease through biomedical research. Scientific discovery begins with the desire to understand what a condition is and what causes it on a molecular and genetic level. Researchers want to find out how it varies among individuals and what factors influence it. We develop tests to reliably identify the condition apart from potentially hundreds of other options with the same signs and symptoms. Biomedical research requires decades of effort, thousands of ideas tried and discarded, a wide variety of people willing to participate in trials, and well-trained scientists whose primary motivation is expanding understanding of how our bodies work and how they break down.

These studies are not sexy,* and they are often years away from any real-world application like creating a medicine to treat a given condition. But long before pharmaceutical companies step in with their deep pockets to test treatments and find cures, biomedical research is underway, and it requires resources. The teams of scientists who conduct this type of work need ten to fifteen years of training to be able to lead research staff, trainees, and students along this journey. This work requires funding that is not driven by profit, because it often takes a long time to make progress and the expected failure-to-success ratio is incompatible with a financially solvent business.

The National Institutes of Health, or the NIH, is the largest biomedical research enterprise in the world, responsible for nearly all major discoveries that support human health and well-being. In 2025, the NIH annual budget was nearly $50 billion. Within the NIH are 27 Institutes and Centers, each with a particular focus. For example, the National Heart, Lung, and Blood Institute supports most cardiovascular and pulmonary research. The National Institute of Diabetes and Digestive and Kidney Diseases produces research on diabetes, kidney, and everything related to the digestive tract. The National Cancer Institute (NCI) has the largest dollar allotment year after year. Before a drug company comes out with an $80,000-per-dose cancer drug that precisely targets the immune system, researchers at the NCI and at universities that receive grants from the NCI have engaged in decades of research to first discover that special target. The NIH and its various institutes are critical to research innovation in health. Where its dollars go, scientific discov-

* Except to the scientists who are oriented and adapted to care a great deal about their tiny slice of discovery on the human condition.

ery follows, and when we learn more, we have more options for treatment and cures.*

As this is a book about the womb, you may be curious about the National Institute of Gynecologic Disease. Or perhaps you'd like to learn about the important work of the National Institute for Women's Health. Unfortunately, neither exists. We do have the National Institute of Child Health and Human Development. That's right. We have *one* institute to cover *all* pediatric health *and* all things related to pregnancy and motherhood. Most women and folks with a uterus spend more than 90 percent of their lives not pregnant. But where are the resources for research focused on the womb unrelated to pregnancy and the rest of the female reproductive organs? The structure and funding of the NIH matches what we already know about how society values women.

Research into reproductive health outside of pregnancy gets folded in anywhere it can find a home. Sometimes it's the National Institute of Child Health and Human Development, because women with gynecologic organs can also be mothers. Sometimes it is the National Institute on Aging, because women do in fact age. Most relevant to my work is the National Cancer Institute, though when petitioning them for funding, I know it's unlikely that an expert on gynecologic cancers will review my proposal. This is disappointing, as only an expert understands our current biomedical landscape as it pertains to gynecologic health and disease. In fact, proposals that are the *least* likely to be funded by the NIH are those that 1) focus on gynecologic disease, 2) focus on health equity topics, and 3) come from underrepresented racial and ethnic minority scientists.

In 2024, less than 7 percent of the entire NIH budget went to study women's health, and the vast majority of this was spent on

* The NIH also features the National Institute of Environmental Health Sciences, focused on how environmental settings, including toxins and pollution, impact health. In fact, in every institute is a through line of research on prevention. This is why discovering the innate mechanism of disease is so critical. It is the gateway to cure but also to prevent what ails us. As of writing this, top scientists at the NIEHS and several other institutes have resigned, as their work is not valued by the current administration, which prizes health propaganda over scientific discovery.

breast cancer and pregnancy research. The reason for such glaring inequity includes a combination of congressional directives on research funding, the NIH leadership's interests, and, as always, the misogyny that regards gynecologic, nonpregnant womb issues as less important.* In 2024, the Biden administration proposed a new initiative to inject funding into the science of women's health, with plans to begin chipping away at the decades of inequitable funding. This was a great first step that was immediately threatened by the November 2024 US presidential election results. Given this deep and ongoing underinvestment in women's health, it is amazing we know what we do about gynecologic health at all. Still, the persistent gaps in knowledge are unacceptable. And even the biomedical research that has focused on women's health has too often led to the exploitation, deception, and harm of Black women specifically.

Black women have significant distrust in research participation, given the historical abuses we have suffered. In the US Public Health Service Untreated Syphilis Study at Tuskegee, government-funded researchers immorally withheld curative treatment from Black people who had acquired syphilis, allowing the disease to ravage their bodies and pass on to their children for decades. In Baltimore, Maryland, just ninety minutes from the nation's capital, a Black woman named Henrietta Lacks sought care for a cervical mass that ended up being cancer. As was routine at the time, her tissue was taken for research purposes and shared with the world without consent. Her tissue cells were unique and had an ability to stay alive and replicate indefinitely. These immortal HeLa cells went on to be crucial in developing the polio and COVID-19 vaccines, understanding how HIV infects the human body, countless cancer research discoveries, and even research in outer space.

I get chills when I think of Ms. Henrietta Lacks and the HeLa cells. The first immortal cells were discovered in a Black woman with a gynecologic cancer. *They came from the Black womb.* No amount of

* In its official report on the state of women's health research, the National Academy of Medicine commented that the NICHD, easily the institute most open to womb research, "focuses primarily on women's health as a mechanism to produce healthy offspring." It is truly stunning.

dry scientific papers will take away the clear and powerful ancestral message of this to me. The Black womb is not broken; it is immensely *strong*. The reason Black women suffer so much from gynecologic disease is because that Womb Strength is used to justify our neglect, while simultaneously being exploited to further biomedical knowledge. Why do I, a woo-woo girl at heart, devote my career to using science to study the womb? Because it's time to tip the scales back in our favor. I am interested in every research question that comes from this perspective: We are not broken; the world has just consistently tried to break us. What does that breaking look like *scientifically*? What does it look like *biologically*? And with that information, *how do we heal*?

MY LOVE OF THE WOMB

As a physician and gynecologic oncologist, I was trained to see the uterus (the womb) as an organ that just follows directions. I learned about the womb as a passive entity that does not produce hormones or tell other organs what to do. But when things go wrong for the womb, nothing else is safe. Everything falls apart. When the womb goes wrong, you can't birth children. When the womb acts up, you spend half the month stuck in the house for fear that your clothes and anything you sit on could be soaked in blood. The womb falls apart and now you face death much earlier than you ever imagined. The womb was never a docile, placid subordinate. Just as women were never that. Just as Black women were *certainly* never that.

I do not devalue the other organs that make up the female reproductive system. The ovaries provide the hormones that influence our wombs and the rest of our bodily functions. They house millions of human eggs, a critical building block of all human life. They too can go wrong. Polycystic ovary syndrome (PCOS) is destabilizing to the usual menstrual cycle and for many people creates symptoms they battle their entire reproductive lives. Ovarian cancer is one of the deadliest cancers a person can face. It often arrives with little warning and requires a treatment journey that is long and too often fails. The fallopian tubes connect the ovaries with the uterus and ferry eggs from the former to the latter. They also act up. They are sometimes inflamed or malformed. They get bloated and create cysts at random. They are very susceptible to infection, and many scientists theorize that the fallopian tubes are the actual originating site of most ovarian cancers. The vulva and the vagina are the gateways to the reproductive system and have their own complex stories. Though these organs and some of their misfortunes will be touched on in these chapters, this book is unapologetically about the womb and the womb alone.

I choose the womb as my focus because it is worth it. I choose the womb because it is enough. I choose the womb because it is often the last story told or left out altogether. The nonpregnant womb, the uterus itself, is almost never mentioned, never part of our public discourse. Yet based on my experiences with my own womb since I was a child, my years of education and training as an aspiring surgeon, my years practicing gynecologic oncology and saving Black women from cancers of the womb, I can tell you the womb matters. The medical and public health communities can no longer afford to neglect the womb, and we as individuals cannot either. As I will argue throughout this book, the womb, more so than any other organ, mirrors the trials and tribulations of being a Black woman in Western society. We ignore and neglect the womb at our peril.

When Black women learn how to silence and compartmentalize our suffering while achieving our goals, we are inheriting a prized skill that was required to survive in this land. The Black enslaved women subjected to endless medical experimentation, rape, and terror at some point learned to stop screaming.* There is a level of control required to do this that I believe I first saw watching my mother sur-

* The towering performance of this by Academy Award–winning actress Lupita Nyong'o in one of the early rape scenes in *12 Years a Slave* has never left me. Devastating suffering—in silence.

vive my father. In the setting of very little external control, she exercised her will through the active suppression of the pain of her struggles. After my school expulsion, I showed up every day to my last-minute summer job in the engineering dean's office to track down alumni and sing the praises of the school that cast me aside when I was no longer excellent. I then took my dejected, ashamed, and depressed self to work in that biomedical engineering research lab, spinning failure into a résumé builder, with no one the wiser. Later, when I sat and endured a public excoriation by my residency training colleagues for the sin of wanting to give back to my community, I did so with stoicism and resolve. As souls inhabiting bodies, here on this spinning third rock from the sun, we simply cannot do this internal smothering without bodily consequences. Silencing is not nuanced. Our bodies and their signals, our voice and its cries for help, get smothered too.

Generations of being underserved and holding low expectations of gynecologic healthcare make Black women incredibly vulnerable to *anyone* who offers solutions for the womb. An untold amount of cultural and ancestral knowledge was wiped out by the violence of the transatlantic slave trade and the colonization and erasure of Indigenous learnings back in our African countries of origin. In the absence of ancestral knowledge, our instinct is to turn to medical professionals to teach us how to care for our bodies in general and our wombs in particular. In the arena of gynecology, though, knowledge is slim due to the limits of women's health research.

So, I see an increasing movement to turn to medicine-adjacent folks, such as wellness influencers who come from a variety of nongynecologic backgrounds and self-described healers whose training is murkily understood at best. There are fantastic, helpful people in this medicine-adjacent space who are giving people the language and tools to improve their relationship to their bodies, and specifically their wombs. They often offer a holistic approach that treats us as full human beings rather than as disembodied problems, which is a welcome change from what we too commonly experience in doctors' offices and hospitals. But they can also offer false solutions based on pseudoscience and vibes, peddling any number of worthless treatments for serious gynecologic diseases. As the most underserved and highly exploited, Black women are especially vulnerable to this secondary harm. I understand why Black women often turn away from science and medicine in their search for healing. My field has left a huge unmet need, and I aim to use these pages to fill the gap.

Gynecology itself is intricately linked to Black womanhood in this country, and with our origin stories, I'm not sure how we would expect to be anywhere but where we are. I hope the information in this book helps you navigate both unregulated spaces and the medical establishment. My goal is to support you in feeling in control of your gynecologic health journey.

Together, let's rethink what it means to be strong.

CHAPTER 3

THE BASICS

Anatomy and Our Reproductive Lives

This book is packed with information and stories with the goal of prompting you to reflect and then act. I suggest taking notes in the margins or in the notes section of your digital reading device while you move through each chapter. Speed-reading will not allow you to fully experience this book. Read and discuss it in community. I will give you clear explanations and an accurate medical vocabulary that you can then use to share your experiences with others as well as communicate your symptoms and conditions to a medical provider. There is a great deal of shame for women and all folks assigned female at birth around their genitals and their reproductive organs and what they should or shouldn't be able to endure. This book is designed to combat that shame. Being comfortable with our bodies begins when we take time to notice them, understand the changes they undergo, and learn how to communicate about those changes. These steps are critical to having a positive and effective gynecologic health journey.

As I reviewed in chapter 1, "Introduction," there are current gaps in the science of understanding each of the four conditions of focus in this book (heavy menstrual bleeding, endometriosis, fibroids, and uterine cancer), largely because the necessary research is chronically underfunded, due to a bias against research that focuses on women, Black people, and health equity. It also doesn't help that thought leaders in public health generally shy away from discussing these conditions and their disproportionate effect on Black women. Thus, we must fill in some of these gaps ourselves, both in understanding patterns that are unique to us and in knowing what types of care to demand. The key to survival is advocating for ourselves and one another. This book is designed to give you this key.

LEARNING THE BASICS: ANATOMY

Anatomy is the first step to knowing how to communicate about our bodies and understand what's normal and what isn't. I'm going to break it down simply here. Later in the book, as we go through each of the four conditions, I will layer on more detail relevant to each disease and your understanding of it.

As a practicing gynecologic oncologist, I drew as I spoke to almost all my new patients. On any piece of paper that we had lying around, I sketched out the gynecologic organs and what, specifically, was going on inside the person's body as we discussed their condition and plans going forward. The most common reaction I received was some variation of "Oh, I have never understood it like that before!" Patients have told me they folded up and carried around their drawing for weeks and longer to remind themselves and help tell others about their conditions. I want to do the same for you here.

In that spirit, these are not slick drawings with every detail but rather a Dr. Doll schematic drawn to communicate the most important information at the level we need to understand it for the conversation we are having.

Figure 1 is our anchor. Let's take a look and move from the outside in. The vagina is the tubular structure that is the middle opening between our legs. It sits beneath our urethra, which leads to the bladder, and above the anus, which leads to the colon. Moving into the vagina and traveling up, we find at the top, where it ends, the cervix.

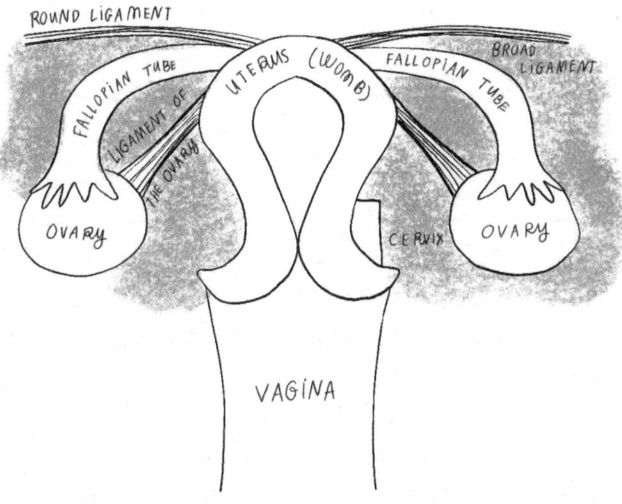

The cervix is part of the uterus. It is not a separate organ. The cervix is the lowest part of the uterus, where the uterine walls fold completely together to form a barrier between the vagina and the inner, protected uterine cavity. When gynecologists use a speculum to open the vaginal walls and look inside, what we see at the end of the vagina is the face of the cervix and the small opening we call the *os*. This view is drawn below, in figure 2.

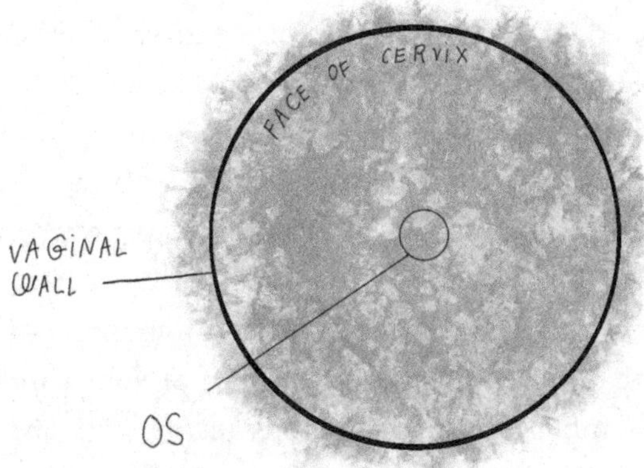

Everything else in figure 1 is hidden inside the body. Let's go there next.

The uterus is a triangle-shaped, fist-size organ with an open cavity in the middle. The wall of the uterus is muscular and thick, while the outer surface is smooth and thin. The inner surface, or the *endometrium,* can be many things. It is the place where a new pregnancy implants and grows, the place where polyps—benign or malignant—can pop up, the place where even a small fibroid can cause lots of problems, and ultimately, the place we bleed from during every menstrual cycle.

Coming off the two upper corners of the uterus are the fallopian tubes. They start off tunneled in the uterine wall, then spread outward with fingerlike edges that drape on the ovaries. These tubes connect the inner cavity of the uterus to the rest of the pelvis. They are soft, fairly fragile, and super stretchy.

At the end of each fallopian tube, we find an ovary. Ovaries are made up of your collection of unfertilized eggs (oocytes), the gland-filled tissue between them, and a thin, clear surface layer that wraps them all together.

A series of ligaments connect these organs to one another and to the body walls. The round ligament holds the top of the uterus in place. The ligament of the ovaries adds support for these small organs, which are otherwise unattached. (Remember: The fallopian tubes drape across them but do not hold them up.) The large, broad ligament then loosely connects the outer surfaces of the uterus, tubes, and ovaries together in the body and to the body wall.

As mentioned, the cervix is part of the uterus. Otherwise, these organs are separate, with distinctly different kinds of tissue, different functions, and different ways things can go wrong. Your eyes, nose, and mouth are all connected on your face but are each very different organs. Think of the gynecologic organs the same way. Connected, but distinct.

When you think about your abdomen and pelvis—the part of your body from your lower ribs to the tops of your thighs—it's important to remember that all the organs inside lay right next to and on top of one another. They each have their own place, but no intervening space. Think of houses so close together that neighbors can high-five one another from their respective windows. It's crowded. This is even more so the case in the pelvis, where the uterus is nestled between the bladder and the colon. These close quarters are drawn in figure 3 below. Cozy.

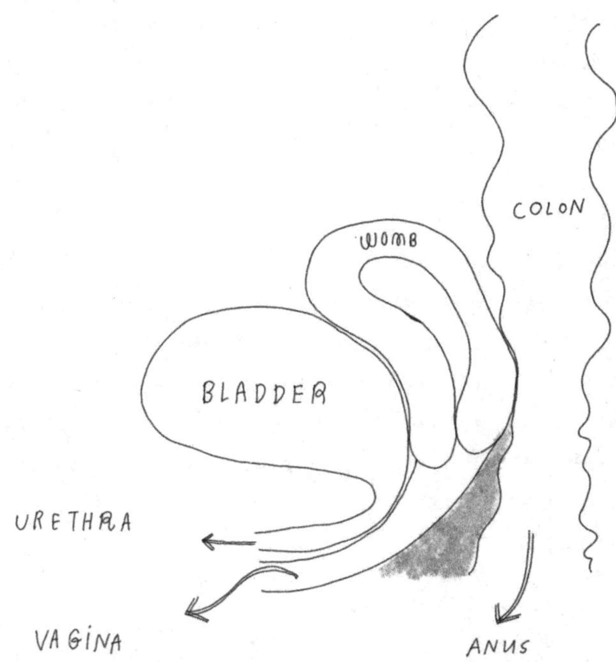

LEARNING THE BASICS: THE GYNECOLOGIC PHASES OF LIFE

One of the coolest things about gynecologic organs is how much they change in function and structure over our lifespans. This is different from nearly every other organ in our bodies. Your heart grows but does the same job from your first breath to your last. Same with your lungs, your kidneys, your stomach, your liver, and so on. Not the gynecologic organs! In each phase of our lives, they are doing very different things.

Let's walk through the phases.

BEFORE THE START OF PERIODS (PREMENARCHE)

In this phase, things are mostly quiet but growing. Though we are born with all the eggs we'll ever have in our ovaries, there is still a great deal of maturation of the eggs and the rest of the ovarian tissue that happens in childhood, during the first ten years or so of life. The uterus, tubes and vagina also grow in size. During these years, in the run-up to *menarche* (the first period), there is some low-level hormonal release from the ovaries. For most of us, this is our most physically androgynous period, during which those assigned female, male, or intersex at birth all look the same, aside from the small real estate between our legs. Ironically, this may also be when some of us felt the most physically free—before the trappings of womanhood began to dictate our relationship to our bodies. During this time, I was a ball of energy and highly accident prone. My default condition was skinned knees, bruised elbows, and knocking over cups, bowls, and dishes at about half of my meals. The only awareness I had of my own reproductive organs was having to sit to pee. But they were there, slowly maturing.

THE FIRST PERIOD (MENARCHE)

Depending on your experience, this may have been exciting, dreadful, or something you don't remember much about. Regardless of its emotional or psychological impact, one's first period is a major event for our bodies. This usually happens between the ages of nine and fifteen. The first period occurs during puberty when signals from the brain (hypothalamus), the pituitary gland, thyroid, ovaries, and adrenal glands prompt the uterus to begin menstruation. It is not uncommon for the first year of cycles to be irregular as the body is learning and maturing the complex feedback loops required for predictable menstruation. My first period was not a surprise to me. I started bleeding at home, on a weekend, when I was twelve. I calmly wiped the blood I saw dripping into the toilet and put on one of the pads from the stash my mother had put in my bathroom the year before. I remember so clearly that I felt sad. After learning about my mother's reproductive trauma and my grandmother's death in childbirth, I now wonder if the sadness I felt was ancestral in a way. I had a few years of being both aware and in control of my body *and* free from the womb and its powerful impact on my family's story. That day, I was initiated into our generational journey.

THE REPRODUCTIVE YEARS

This is the phase where our gynecologic organs are involved in a monthly orchestration designed around the *potential* for pregnancy during each given cycle. It's helpful to remember that before the advent and availability of medical contraception, when all we had were barrier methods (i.e., condoms), withdrawal, and ovulation timing to prevent pregnancy, women and all folks with a uterus had more pregnancies. A lot more. During pregnancy and frequent breastfeeding, ovulation is suppressed and the monthly menstrual cycle is shut off. A single pregnancy can mean one to two years without ovulating. This means our ancestors, both recent and distant, had *significantly fewer menstrual cycles in their lifetimes* than what we currently experience. To give you a numerical sense, one estimate is that, in 1919, women had an average of forty menstrual cycles in their lifetime. That number is now four hundred. This is an important idea to keep in mind as we move through various treatment strategies I cover in this book, some of which involve menstrual cycle suppression.

From the ages of twelve to twenty-two, I had a cycle every single month. It was painful, heavy, embarrassing, and a complete inconvenience. I bled through my pants while taking physics exams. I cramped so terribly I would walk around semi–bent over until the pain medication kicked in. One summer in college, while riding the A train in hot New York City through the infamously long stretch between 59th and 125th Streets, I passed such a large clot that I could feel the blood sliding down my leg. I ran off the train at 168th Street and begged a local bodega owner (in barely adequate Spanish) to use their bathroom to change into the new pads I had just purchased. I had no internal visualization of what my cycle was other than a deluge of pain and suffering. I resented the womb for existing at all, without knowing anything about it other than the blood. I wish now that I had known what I'm about to describe in the next section—what is actually happening inside.

What is menstruation from a physiological standpoint? I recognize menstruation has cultural implications and can represent much more than what's happening in the body. However, if we don't also understand the biology, we are left at a great disadvantage in navigating our gynecologic health. The reproductive phase of a person's life usually lasts thirty to fifty years. We deserve to understand it.

The womb exists on a cyclical clock from the onset of puberty to a person's last period. That clock is controlled by hormones from the ovaries and kickoff signals from the brain, which together create a well-orchestrated symphony. If the ovaries and brain play the tune, then the womb is the dancer, growing a lush layer of blood vessels, tissue, and scaffolding in tune to the music, and shedding the very same layer when the music stops. That shedding is what we call a *period*—or *menstruation*—and it announces itself with the onset of vaginal bleeding every twenty-four to thirty-eight days. There are many ways to explain the menstrual cycle, and I prefer those that put the focus on bleeding as the center of the cycle, rather than ovulation. It's the bleeding we notice most anyway.

Figure 4 is the overview of this perspective. The two primary hormones produced in the ovaries are estrogen and progesterone.* Here is what they do: In general, estrogen promotes the growth of the *endometrium,* the inner lining of the uterus. New endometrial glands

* There are many types of each. For the purpose of the menstrual cycle and this book, I am almost always referring to 17beta-estradiol (E2), and pregn-4-ene-3,20-dione (P4). In addition, there's a convention of using *estradiol* and *progestins* when speaking of external medication and *estrogen* and *progesterone* when referring to the internal molecules. I will primarily use *estrogen* and *progesterone* throughout for simplicity.

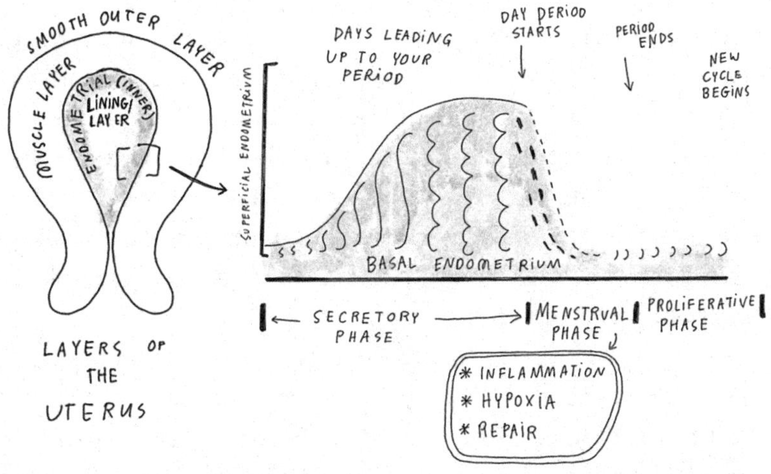

and the tissue they live in grow and thicken in response to estrogen. This is called the *proliferative phase* of the endometrium, because the endometrial tissue is proliferating, or growing. While this is happening, an egg cell in the ovaries is maturing and starting to produce our second main hormonal player, progesterone. As this egg fully matures, progesterone levels rise. The rise of progesterone creates two important effects: 1) It blocks the estrogen effect—estrogen levels fall, and the endometrium stops growing; 2) it prompts the endometrium to shift from growing into maturing. This maturation is called the *secretory phase*. The endometrium's newly formed basic blood vessels now arch into spiral patterns, connect to one another via delicate capillaries, and wrap themselves in smooth muscle that can contract and relax, regulating blood flow. This endometrium, made up of glands, complex vasculature, and an extracellular tissue matrix holding it all together, is now ready for a potential pregnancy or, much more commonly, menstruation.*

* If you've read blogs, watched videos, or searched images of menstruation, you've likely encountered the terms *follicular phase* and *luteal phase* of the cycle. These are referencing the activity in the ovaries and a way to describe the cycle focused on *ovulation*. I have chosen to describe the cycle rooted in what is happening in the womb; however, the follicular phase of the ovary roughly corresponds to the proliferative phase of the endometrium, while the luteal phase of the ovary corresponds to the secretory phase of the endometrium.

When there is no pregnancy, bleeding is triggered by the sudden fall in progesterone levels. This marks entry to the *menstrual phase*. A simple way to think about it is if progesterone is keeping the lights on—in this case, the lights being the mature endometrium—once the progesterone is gone, the lights turn off, and the mature endometrium sheds. A singular event then occurs, and it's one that happens nowhere else in the body: a recurring wounded surface that heals without a scar, over and over and over again. If you want to hear more detail about that, read on.*

To start, I need to tell you a bit more about the endometrium. While it is just one of the layers of the full uterine wall, the endometrium itself is made of its own two layers. The upper two-thirds of the endometrium is the superficial layer, and the lower third is the basal layer. It's the superficial layer that sheds during menstruation. The basal layer is attached to the underlying uterine muscle wall and stays in place.† So falling progesterone levels trigger the *menstrual phase,* but how? The answer is a series of three events: inflammation, hypoxia (oxygen restriction), and finally, repair. Inflammation in this case is healthy and necessary. The inflammation brings in molecules called *prostaglandins* and other factors that cause the endometrium to break down. Specifically, prostaglandins create holes in the walls of the endometrial vessels that become leaky and ooze blood. The prostaglandins also cause edema (tissue swelling) and attract more inflammatory cells and enzymes that cause tissue breakdown. In summary, the vessels are leaky and bleeding, the inflammatory cells and enzymes cause edema and tissue breakdown, and eventually, you start to bleed.‡ Your period has started.

---

* You certainly don't need to know the details of the menstrual event to advocate for your gynecologic health, but I think it's worth understanding so we can demystify what is happening in the body when one person bleeds for four days and another for four months.

† This will become very relevant when we dive into treatments for heavy bleeding and fibroids (chapters 4 and 6) and endometrial cancer (chapter 7).

‡ This inflammatory breakdown starts a few days before you see the first drop of blood with your period—in case you were wondering why that "late luteal phase" can feel heavy and slow and emotional. It's actually the start of the *menstrual phase.*

How does it end? This part is impressive. The very same factors that create this inflammatory cascade also deliver the ingredients for its resolution. The prostaglandin causes leaky vessels but also stimulates the smooth muscle cells on the blood vessels to contract, limiting the amount of blood lost. The loss of blood and the vessel wall contraction create a low-oxygen environment—hypoxia—which the body responds to automatically by sending blood-clotting factors that start to quench the flow of blood. Macrophages, which rushed in with the inflammation, are cells that eat up the debris and remains of the endometrial tissue that has just been destroyed. In other words, the cleanup crew comes in right alongside the inflammation cascade and starts wrapping things up. The bleeding stops. And the basal endometrial layer, that lower third, remains untouched and capable of regeneration. As the ovaries restart their clock, estrogen levels start to rise. Endometrial stem cells begin rebuilding the tissue and vessels. The cycle begins again. A wound with a scarless repair.*

People tell me their periods are sensitive to changes in their life, stress being a common one. I think, *Of course.* Your immune system is sensitive to chronic or acute stress,† and so a process tied to a robust and healthy physiologic immune response is going to be sensitive too. If the brain kickoff signals that control ovulation are off-kilter one month, that means the estrogen-and-progesterone dance is off too, and here comes a "weird" or irregular cycle. Fluctuations in the menstrual cycle are normal and expected. One random short cycle or one month where bleeding lasts an extra day can happen and is part of healthy cycle variation. But this book is not about healthy cycle

The tissue in your womb is literally, rapidly, deconstructing in real time. So, take it easy.

* By the way, we used to think that vessels grew completely new, each month. Now we know that what they do is much more complicated and magical. They regrow from fragments of old vessels, they sprout off new branches, and they coalesce multiple broken vessels into new ones. They regenerate, holding on to pieces from the last cycle. How's that for the symbolism of the womb?

† Anybody else get sick every college semester after exam week?

variation. It's about chronically abnormal menstruation, heavy bleeding, terrible pelvic pain, and cancerous growths, all of which can, if we're not vigilant, be mistaken as normal and cause great harm.

My goal is to help you identify these more serious aberrations and take action to heal.

I did not lose touch with my femininity, my natural rhythms, or my intuition when I began using gynecologic treatments to ease my Womb Suffering. The opposite happened—I got *more* in touch with my body, now having a responsibility to track how each treatment was or was not working, noticing my patterns over long stretches of time. I got *more* in touch with my femininity and my intuition because I no longer engaged in the nonspecific blanket suppression of physical and emotional signals that came alongside my Womb Suffering. When we live under conditions of intergenerational oppression, sexual violence, and the exploitation of the Black body, what is "naturally" occurring to us every month may not be what we were designed to inherit. I respect deeply the emotional, spiritual, and ancestral power of the womb—and I do not believe I was born to suffer.

PERIMENOPAUSE AND MENOPAUSE

Technically, perimenopause is when the ovarian hormonal signals start to decline and menstrual cycles start to space out. A whole host of other downstream effects hit us as these two events happen. The organs themselves undergo change. As growth signals decline, the ovaries get smaller, often to the point where they may no longer be seen on routine imaging studies. There is a much lower chance for pregnancy and fewer cycles of inflammation and repair, and so the uterus is no longer changing drastically in size. The cervix appears smaller and paler, with a smaller and smaller opening. The vaginal walls also lose some elasticity and lubrication as hormonal levels drop.

Regarding bleeding, the early signs of entering the menopausal transition is when periods are seven or more days "late," consistently.

The cycles are spreading out more and more. And, on average, once your bleeding cycles become greater than sixty days apart and you are in the most common decade of menopause (forty-five to fifty-five), this usually indicates being in the final year of natural bleeding in your life. Other folks who have surgery to remove their ovaries will go through what we call *surgical menopause,* regardless of their age.*

In Black women, perimenopausal symptoms have been noted to start earlier and last longer. From a gynecologist's viewpoint, the perimenopause phase is a time when menstrual bleeding is still occurring, and new menopausal symptoms have started, such as hot flashes, mood swings, vaginal dryness, and palpitations. We then think of the menopause phase as the full cessation of all menstruation (periods) *even if other menopausal symptoms are still active.* This is traditionally defined as twelve months without a period. However, the cacophony of voices on social media defines *menopause* in other ways. This lack of agreement around the term can lead to confusion as people attempt to share their symptoms with their doctors.

Over the years in treating patients with gynecologic cancers and countless conversations with my oncology colleagues, we all share the same stories of Black women with a new cancer diagnosis telling us, "Well, my period never stopped. I never stopped bleeding." I worry that even the way I have described menopause here is missing crucial nuance from Black women's experiences that have been continually under-researched. I wonder if, for Black women and perhaps all minoritized folks subjected to intergenerational oppression, we need to deprioritize the criteria of "no bleeding for twelve months" and focus instead on the onset of menopausal symptoms and their severity when defining a Black woman as "menopausal."

As you continue to read about what's normal, what's abnormal, and what is clear evidence of gynecologic disease, keep in mind that "menopausal" means that the monthly menstrual cycles are finished.

* Research from Dr. Maya Wright, a Black woman and PhD student at the time, demonstrated that although initially the rate of surgical menopause was higher in White women, as of 2014, at least in the state of North Carolina, rates were increasing and are now higher among Black women.

Things are quieter, but these organs are still *there*. Our awareness of this and our attention to our bodies during late perimenopause and full menopause can be lifesaving.

This is our anatomy and the phases of our gynecologic life story and concludes part 1, "How We Begin." In part 2, "How We Live," we will take an in-depth look at the four conditions of the womb: heavy bleeding, endometriosis, fibroids, and endometrial (uterine) cancer. Over the course of four chapters and the intimate accounts of people who have battled these health challenges, we will discover how things go wrong, and how we, as Black women in particular, have been taught to endure while shining bright and breaking barriers.

A NOTE ON THE GLOSSARY

Despite my attempt to use as little medical jargon as possible, I still include words and phrases in this book that I hope you will come to know and become comfortable using. I'm motivated to give you the right language to advocate for yourself and not feel talked over simply because you are unfamiliar with certain words. To that end, this book contains a glossary of commonly and not-so-commonly used terms from biology and medicine as reference as you read and beyond as you take control of your gynecologic health journey.

Part II

HOW WE LIVE

The Four Conditions of the Womb

CHAPTER 4

HEAVY MENSTRUAL BLEEDING

The Suffering Womb

I remember when my period came during a week of dance performances. We were to be in white tutus and light pink tights. I knew my typical fix for dance class—doubling the sanitary pads in my leotard—wouldn't fly. I was thirteen and anxious. When I asked my mother what to do, she had no advice to give me. In her mind, using a tampon was akin to losing your virginity. I went into those performances robbed of my excitement. All I felt was the terror of bleeding onstage, and so I struggled mightily to dance as if nothing was amiss, clenching all the wrong muscles while trying to move gracefully. When I wasn't dancing, I stood in the bathroom watching my mother scrub stains out of my white tutu costume in between performances over and over that weekend. I learned then what we do with the blood. We pretend it doesn't exist, we perform as if we are not in pain, and we clean up behind closed doors.

Even as a girl, my womb was already a place of suffering. My mother could be harsh, but those days when I was laid out in bed, moaning with cramps, were often when I

found the most tenderness from her. She would offer few words but would pat my back and feed me painkillers. And so the womb was also, indirectly, a place of comfort, a mystery that held both misery and balm.

Dr. Whitney Ragan Robinson has been my friend and scientific collaborator for over ten years. We met when I was starting my research training, after completing my OB-GYN residency and the first half of my gynecologic oncology fellowship. I had just enrolled in graduate school, and she was an early-career assistant professor in the Department of Epidemiology at the University of North Carolina at Chapel Hill. Her educational pedigree was beyond impressive. Coming out of public schools in Memphis, Tennessee, she earned admission to Harvard University, graduating with a degree in biochemical sciences and going on to complete her PhD in epidemiology.

Our first meeting had been something of a blind work date. I was in my second year of gynecologic oncology fellowship. I had been making noise to my mentors about wanting to access multi-hospital data to study gynecologic cancer care patterns across the state. Whitney had been making noise to her colleagues about wanting to study the connection between race and hysterectomy patterns across the state. I needed her epidemiological background to help me design rigorous studies. She needed my clinical background to help find and interpret the relevant information amid thousands of billing records and medical claims. As two Black women academics in a predominantly White institution, we also simply needed each other. It was a match made in heaven. We went on to successfully partner on several small research grants that led to larger projects and research findings that have changed practice in gynecology.* Our collaborations con-

* The Carolina Hysterectomy Cohort is one such result. Led by Whitney, this is a massive dataset of every hysterectomy across ten hospitals and hundreds of outpatient clinics in North Carolina. Our work using this research is covered in chapters 5 and 6. I subsequently led the process to leverage this cohort, and expand it, to challenge a major racial quality of care gap in endometrial cancer diagnosis, covered in detail in chapter 7.

tinue in full force to this day, as does our friendship. We took a girls' trip to the Essence Festival of Culture in 2018, and she joined me in Seattle, Washington, for my multiday fortieth birthday celebration in 2022. And yet, when we sit down on a Friday in the summer of 2024, I have a feeling I will learn things about my friend that have never come out in our time together. We've spent hundreds of hours talking about gynecologic health and disease in the data and very little about our own experiences.

Whitney is wearing a new KAMALA T-shirt and sitting with a familiar backdrop—a room in her house where I can hear the sounds of her young boys playing (and sometimes screaming) in the background. She has natural hair in a braided style that makes me imagine a young Black girl, between her mother's knees, getting a swoop of cornrows that end in a side fall of soft short twists. Whitney's family is Black American, with deep roots in the US South. Many generations back, her maternal ancestors settled in Alabama where her grandmother and then her mother were raised. I have always felt a gravity in Whitney's presence, and today, I wonder if it's because she embodies the unbroken line of Black women who survived the unimaginable—kidnapping, being carried like cargo across an ocean, enslavement, rape, and unending psychological violence—and are still here. What are the epigenetic signatures she carries with her right alongside the powerful cultural legacy?

Whitney describes her mother as being extremely hardworking and entirely practical. She had a strong sense of right and wrong and was unafraid to share it. Her mother also had a perfectionist streak, and one of the things she wanted to do perfectly was parent. Although Whitney's softer and more sensitive take on the world could clash painfully with her mother's directness, I can tell she clearly respects and appreciates all that her mother imparted to her. This gratitude includes that deep practicality (and minimal emotion) with which she approached teaching her only daughter about how to care for herself when she started her periods.

Whitney's first period occurred when she was ten years old. She had been in bed sleeping with her mom, because her father was out of town and it was still a practice that brought Whitney comfort. She woke up to go to the bathroom and discovered blood in her underwear. "My mother must have told me something about it before, because I remember I was not shocked. I just came back to tell her what happened and to ask her what to do." Her mother was matter-of-fact in teaching her about using pads and keeping a monthly calendar. Her mother tracked her own cycles on a big wall calendar that was used to organize all family activities. There was a *P* for the day her mother's cycle was expected, and it would then be struck through with an *X* the day it arrived. It was out in the open, next to any assortment of kids' appointments, work meetings, and family trips. And there was no shame. When Whitney entered this arena with her first cycle, a *WP* was added to the calendar. She started carrying a small purse to school to hold her maxi pads, using the calendar to prepare, and following the directions she was taught to keep herself tidy. Her periods were not a problem.

Except for the bleeding.

"I feel like I was pretty regular from the beginning, and looking back, they were heavy," Whitney tells me. "But, like, my mom also had heavy periods, so I think that was normalized. It wasn't a *problem;* it was more a *pain.* I can remember visiting my grandmother for Christmas and I bled through the sheets one night. And my grandmother woke me up, we changed the sheets, you know. . . . And that was not uncommon that I would bleed into my sheets."

Her mother taught her to lay towels on her bed to avoid bleeding accidents. And when she bled through those, they used a special spray to get the stains out. They would check her mattress pad to see if the blood had seeped through that layer as well. They always kept an extra set of sheets on hand and knew to expect more laundry some weeks. All of this was normal to Whitney the child, Whitney the young adult in college and graduate school, and even Whitney the wife and mother. It would be a long time before Whitney the forty-four-year-old expert in the symptom severity of gynecologic conditions could see the problem. By this time, she had already had a hysterectomy.

So, what really counts as "heavy bleeding," as Whitney and so many of us casually say? There is a formal definition, and it may surprise you. I know it surprised me.

Heavy menstrual bleeding—or *menorrhagia,* as it was called for a long time in gynecology—is defined by the National Institute for Health and Care Excellence as "menstrual blood loss of sufficient volume to adversely affect physical, emotional, social and/or material quality of life." I think this definition is one of the primary reasons why Black women are so deeply underdiagnosed. Menorrhagia is inherently subjective. It depends on your own assessment of what blood volume loss is acceptable and, most crucially, what quality of life you should expect.* Surviving Black womanhood in this country requires strength, and modern gynecology has repeatedly shown a lack of empathy for the Black body. It is entirely rational that Black women would have a markedly different understanding of what constitutes a tolerable quality of life.

When I was in gynecology training, I was taught to screen for heavy menstrual bleeding by asking about bleeding that lasts more than seven days in a single cycle; soaking through more than one heavy pad or tampon an hour for more than three hours; or having more than three days of heavy bleeding within a single cycle. When I would use these questions to screen for abnormal bleeding in Black women patients, they often scoffed at me. To them, these were features of a normal cycle. In the moment, I felt silly creating what then felt like false alarm. And then they shared stories of having to use adult diapers or Depends garments to manage bleeding because commercially sold heavy pads were woefully inadequate. They told me about lining trash bags under their bedsheets to save the mattress, because even the thickest diaper or pad could not contain the heaviness of their flow. But they were functioning, they were living, and to the definition I had been taught in medicine, they weren't suffering.

A patient I'll never forget exemplified this pattern of Black women accommodating the suffering. During a routine Pap smear appoint-

* There are normalizing parameters around cycle length, flow, and other characteristics that I go over in detail in part 3, chapter 9.

ment at the Stroger Cook County hospital, when I was in residency training, she told me that her blood flow was so heavy, she went through ten heavy pads a day. I immediately ordered blood work. Her blood level came back as critically and severely anemic—a hemoglobin level of 4 g/dL—which called for immediate hospitalization and blood transfusion. I called her, frantic, but she laughed. "I feel fine. I'm tired sometimes, but who isn't?" she responded. Plus, her family always had "strong" periods, and she couldn't miss work. I was stunned. It turned out she was a grocery store stocker. A physically intensive job that she performed with minimal oxygen-carrying capacity in her blood. If she could do this work at her current levels, what could she do at normal levels? Become an Olympian?! I am ashamed now that all I could initially see was her strength. It was several days later that I also thought about how precarious her life was. For example, if she were in a car accident, losing just a small amount of blood could put her into cardiac arrest, killing her before help could arrive. In a case like that, the autopsy report would say that she hemorrhaged to death—a typical occurrence in an accident. There would be no evidence of the medical invisibility that allowed her anemia to go untreated. And even without the bad luck of a terrible accident, her routine next period could be the tipping point, where she lost enough blood to have dangerously low blood pressures, landing her in an Emergency Department, requiring blood transfusions, time off work, and the cascade of inconveniences that have serious financial and social consequences. She is not alone. In a study of young Black women from Chicago who were not actively seeking gynecologic care for any reason, over one-third (35 percent) who reported having "heavy periods" were clinically anemic by blood test. One in three.

Heavy menstrual bleeding is common. It's the reason for up to 30 percent of all gynecology visits, and depending on who and how you ask, could be as common as affecting 50 percent of women at some point in their lives. It is the reason for half of all hysterectomies in the

United States.* And yet, the condition is severely underdiagnosed. A study of over fifteen thousand women in five countries, including the United States and Canada, found that over six thousand respondents had signs of heavy bleeding, and the average age it started was twenty-six years old.† Here is what else they found:

- 80 percent of the women were worried about bleeding-related accidents
- 70 percent avoided social activities because of their heavy periods
- 40 percent had experienced embarrassing situations related to heavy bleeding
- 69 percent had blood clots with their cycles
- 68 percent had to change their pads more frequently than every two hours to avoid accidents
- 64 percent reported tiredness

These are incredibly symptomatic women with very heavy bleeding. Yet on average from the time their symptoms started, they took three years to act.‡ Most of them first looked for information online and discussed it with friends and family. More than a third decided to just manage it themselves. Less than half ever reported their heavy bleeding to a doctor. And for those who did, the visit rarely went well. Only 34 percent of these women received *any* treatment for their heavy bleeding. This is terrible. It's a statistic that is an indictment on my field. This makes me angry, because treatments really do

---

* Among surgeries that are not done for cancer reasons.

† This varied, though. Of women with HMB, 273 (27.3 percent) had it from a young age; for 219 (21.9 percent), it started after switching or ending contraception; for 238 (23.8 percent), it started postpartum; and for 223 (22.3 percent), the onset of HMB was perimenopausal. The rest (47 women, 4.7 percent) could not be organized into one of the predefined categories.

‡ In my research, we call this the *appraisal interval*—a major factor that influences delay to healthcare. It's the time between when you have a symptom and when you perceive there's a reason to go get it checked out. Three years is a very, very long appraisal interval.

work. In fact, for women who were treated in this study, *most* had their bleeding get better and reported successful symptom relief without surgery.

Heavy menstrual bleeding can be a problem across all women and folks with a uterus, but it is much worse for those who are also Black in this country. For us, it doesn't start with that first time you may tell a doctor that your periods are heavy. Instead, all too often, it starts with powerful negative experiences that shape our entire view of where to go for help. Whitney's story is no different.

Whitney was eighteen years old when she had her first gynecology visit. She was about to go off to college at Harvard University, and she was the first in her family to attend an Ivy League institution. Her mother, always conscientious, scheduled her to see her gynecologist as an item to check off the to-do list. Whitney didn't particularly want to go and was not sexually active, though she is not sure her mother believed her. Her mother's perspective, she tells me, was "this is what we do. This is taking good care of you." She went. The White woman gynecologist performed a vaginal exam. Whitney can't remember whether the doctor had asked if she was sexually active or if she was asked and simply not believed. It is not common practice for a teenager who is not sexually active to be given an internal exam unless there is a specific concern that needs to be investigated. "It wasn't a pleasant experience, but not super traumatic," Whitney summarizes. I get the message and move on. Her brevity indicates to me that she does not want to dwell on this particular memory.

After college, Whitney went to graduate school to study epidemiology. Doing so fed her aptitude for numbers, the scientific process, and health equity. She was drawn to learn more about reproductive health and cancer, and she noticed how little was known about these conditions in Black people specifically. I smile as she speaks, because we share this motivation around using our perspective and skills to improve the quality of research on Black people's health. "As a graduate student, I was literally reading the scientific literature, and I'm like, everything they're saying here is wrong," she recalls. Her perception from early on was that the problems that occur in Black communities were being badly investigated by White researchers. She was motivated to change this.

During this time, in the late 2000s, the human papillomavirus (HPV) vaccine was introduced. Based on Whitney's scientific interests and desire to maintain her own health, she wanted to get the vaccine to prevent cervical cancer and other HPV-related diseases—exactly what the vaccine was developed to do.* She was older than the upper limit of the original age of approval (twenty-six years) and was perfectly happy to pay out of pocket to get it. She knew the HPV vaccine was most effective for those who get it before any sexual intercourse, and she was in that category, regardless of age. She visited the campus gynecologist—a White woman—and filled out the intake form, noting her sexual activity history ("None") alongside her medical information. Again, however, Whitney had an internal pelvic exam performed. This was yet another unnecessary exam my friend had to endure. This time, Whitney tells me more.

Whitney gritted through the uncomfortable exam. Afterward, the gynecologist asked her, "Is your partner very small?" *What?* Whitney repeated what she had already written on the intake sheet: She didn't have a partner; she'd never been sexually active. "Oh," the doctor said. "I would have used a smaller speculum if I had known." At this point in the visit, Whitney cried. "I felt really violated, and I felt like, why are you making all these assumptions about me? Why do I fill out all this stupid paperwork if you're not going to even read it?" I listen, nodding vigorously and wanting to scream, but I don't want to interrupt my friend as she continues the story. The campus gynecologist then suggested that Whitney see a different provider next time who was "known to be gentle." The comment suggested that Whitney, a five-foot-ten-inch-tall Black woman with a solid frame, didn't inspire gentleness in the doctor simply by virtue of being a human being. To this doctor, it seemed that Whitney couldn't possibly be virginal. There was no way she could be negatively affected by a large speculum

* Chiefly genital warts, but also head and neck cancers, respiratory polyps, and vulvar and vaginal cancers.

used during a questionable exam.* To make it worse, Whitney's key needs were not addressed during the appointment. The doctor initiated no discussion, screening, or evaluation for Whitney's heavy menstrual cycles. Whitney wanted the HPV vaccine because she had learned enough to know it was good for her health. What she got was violation. Whitney would return to complete her HPV vaccination series, while otherwise avoiding the gynecology team. She moved on with her professional life, graduating with her PhD and completing a postdoctoral research fellowship at the University of Michigan. And she met her future husband, Louis.

Like most of us, my friend's life didn't stop because of terrible gynecologic care. One way I think Black women suffer for so long from womb conditions is that we can simply adapt to startling levels of pain and fatigue. It is the fatigue, especially, that is dangerously misdiagnosed as simply being "tired." Lack of sleep can make you tired. But so can lack of oxygen, which many of us are silently suffering from. It starts with our cells.

Red blood cells move throughout our bodies, and iron is the micronutrient that carries oxygen in those cells. Iron has other critical roles, including mitochondrial energy metabolism, support for cardiac and skeletal muscle activity, neurotransmitter production, and healthy immune system function. Your endocrine, neurological, musculoskeletal, and immune systems are all impacted by iron. Maintaining the appropriate levels is important.

The problem is that many of us walk around iron deficient. There are three ways this happens: 1) We don't take in enough iron in our diets or supplements; 2) we eat enough iron but we don't absorb enough of it; or 3) we eat and absorb enough iron, but we lose it too quickly—for example, by bleeding too much. Low iron is the most common micronutrient deficiency in the world, precisely because it is often caused by heavy menstrual bleeding. Here is what happens when we don't have enough iron:

* The question of when a pelvic exam should and shouldn't be done is a debated topic, and I have a strong and potentially unpopular opinion. We'll get to that in part 3.

- Step 1: Our bodies pull iron from our iron storage, which is called *ferritin*. When blood tests reveal that iron storage levels / ferritin have dropped too low, this is called *iron deficiency*. Your red blood cell count can be normal, but your iron storage level (ferritin) is low. Normal ferritin level is reported as 10–180 µg/L for most labs, but this is misleading. Symptoms can start when ferritin drops below 50 µg/L, and we have evidence that supplementation starting at this level is helpful.*
- Step 2: With iron storage (ferritin) depleted, our bodies prioritize using the little iron we have left to carry oxygen in those critical red blood cells that circulate around the body. This makes sense because without iron, those red blood cells would die, and without them, we die. But enzymes and proteins in other important system functions do not receive the iron they need. We start to feel this through increasing fatigue and other symptoms.
- Step 3: Eventually, we have so little iron that we don't have enough to even keep the red blood cells going. Their numbers decline, and now we lack enough red blood cells to oxygenate our bodies. We have now reached iron-deficiency anemia, where our red blood cell levels drop below normal. This is measured by our *hemoglobin* (or *hematocrit*) levels. Normal hemoglobin levels are generally 12–15 g/dL.

Iron deficiency is no joke. It impacts mental and physical health and can result in cognitive impairment, fatigue, exhaustion, brain fog, muscle weakness, shortness of breath, dizziness, pica, insomnia, restless leg, and even hair loss.† Remember, at this stage, someone experiencing iron deficiency (step 1 and step 2 above) will still have a "normal" red blood cell (*hemoglobin*) lab test. Yet they can have the same symptoms as someone with severe anemia. Women with iron

* Some labs will report the units as *ng/dL,* which is a 1:1 equivalent to µg/L. They are the same level, just reported differently.

† Yes, hair! Iron deficiency can cause hair thinning and hair loss. If you experience either of these, run—don't walk—to get your levels checked.

deficiency report lower quality of life, low quality of their work, and more missed days at work. I know Black women who were absolute shining stars in their careers while severely iron deficient. Can you imagine what they could do with normal, healthy iron levels?

I was one of these women exhibiting this terrible strength that Black women have. On May 7, 2021, my ferritin (iron storage) level was checked. At this time, I was a practicing gynecologic oncologist conducting long, complex surgeries, I led a multimillion-dollar endometrial cancer research program, I was president of a national nonprofit organization I co-founded, I ran a coaching and consulting business, and I was an emotionally present mother of a six-year-old and a two-year-old. I had my iron checked not because I was feeling tired but because I was losing my hair and didn't understand why.* I went to see Dr. Margaret Towolawi, a Seattle-area Black primary care doctor with an interest in skin and hair conditions for women of color. She insisted we check my iron levels. My results came back: My ferritin was 6 µg/L. I was stunned. My red blood cell count was in the low-normal range, but my iron storage was nearly zero. I was scheduled for a series of IV iron infusions and got to experience firsthand the difference between being depleted and replenished in terms of this essential micronutrient. It was night and day. I now take a daily iron supplement and check my ferritin levels twice a year to be sure this doesn't ever happen to me again.†

As a physician, I no longer use the term *mild anemia,* which is typically used to indicate a red blood cell (hemoglobin) level that is below the normal threshold but not low enough to warrant immediate blood transfusion. What is mild about being at the final stage of a critical micronutrient deficiency? Even in its mildest form, suffering is built into anemia as a diagnosis.

* So, when we get to part 3 of this book and I start lecturing on how we can barely even feel our bodies and our wombs secondary to our overwork and this Terrible Strength, please know that I am very much part of "we," and this healing is what we are all going to do together.

† My iron deficiency was not from heavy bleeding, thankfully. I had an absorption issue, which has improved. And by this point, I had my quota of womb issues, which I'll share more about in the next two chapters.

What does this have to do with the womb? Heavy menstrual bleeding, iron deficiency, and iron-deficiency anemia are deeply interrelated, underreported, and undertreated.* This trifecta is a perfect example of the detrimental impact of silencing around Womb Suffering. Menstrual bleeding is a normal part of female physiology, but our culture demands that it be hidden. Successful femininity is having a period that no one knows about. For Black women, the normalization of heavy bleeding teaches us that suffering silently is a virtue—and that suffering is multifaceted. In one way, we suffer passively, when too much blood leaves the body, and fatigue and the many other symptoms of iron loss set in. In another way, we suffer actively, with the cramping and physical tension that period pain often creates. Then we also suffer from the limitations we live within, restricting our clothing choices, our exercise, and, ultimately, our life experiences when we won't leave the house for days or sometimes weeks at a time. And for those of us who are severely anemic, we may not even be aware of how limited our physical function has become, as we are able to do less and less year after year. We can literally be bleeding to death while no one notices.

It turns out, while my friend Whitney was excelling in her burgeoning career, passing major life milestones, and bleeding every month, she had been told she was "borderline anemic" and could consider taking iron supplements. No healthcare provider investigated the cause of her anemia. What would drive her back to seeking gynecologic care was something else entirely: She'd met Louis, the man who would become her husband. By then, she was in her mid-thirties and had a clear perspective on family planning. My friend's chest expands as she declares, "I firmly believe in multiple layers of birth control. I told him we need at least five methods!" *Amen.* I could relate completely. As a high-achieving Black woman on track for a successful

* One group of researchers trying hard to raise the profile on this issue suggest a memorable phrase: "If you see HMB, think ID!" (ID = iron deficiency)

career, having an unexpected pregnancy was not an option. We were taught it would derail your life and tie you to someone unlikely to be a part of your future happiness. It was a deeply planted fear. So, when Whitney developed a serious relationship with a boyfriend who seemed like he could become more, she once again sought out gynecologic care. This time, she spent energy looking for a caring, thoughtful gynecologist who would see her in her full humanity. She found one, and we'll call her Dr. Smith.

Whitney waited months for the appointment, and then hours in the waiting room for Dr. Smith, who was known to run late because she truly spent time with each patient. After discussing Whitney's desire for contraception, Dr. Smith prescribed a low-dose progestin (progesterone) medication. As I listen intently, I can tell where this story is going. These medications are notorious for causing irregular bleeding. Why would someone prescribe a medication that is almost certain to cause irregular bleeding to a person with a two-decade history of heavy cycles? Whitney started the progestin medication for birth control and immediately started having what she said felt like *daily* irregular bleeding.

After experiencing months of frustration and inconvenience, she called Dr. Smith's office for help. A nurse reassured her it could take up to three months for the bleeding to "even out." Whitney responded that it had been five months already, but her concerns were not taken seriously. Frustrated but not defeated, Whitney tried to help herself. Holding on to her mother's teaching from early years, Whitney started tracking her cycles again and realized she was not bleeding every day but essentially was having a cycle every two weeks.* Armed with this information, she went to Google to look up her medication and read about her change in bleeding pattern. She learned that she was experiencing a hallmark sign of what we call

* This is a really common memory distortion when it comes to bleeding. It is such a disruptive symptom that bleeding for two days in a week where you don't expect it feels like every day. When your plans are disrupted, the impact *is* every day. But this is also why carefully tracking your bleeding can be helpful—because the actual pattern can help a trained provider distinguish the cause.

breakthrough bleeding, where the endometrium begins to shed while it's still in its building (or proliferative) phase.*

She called back armed with the right vocabulary. "I told them, 'I am having breakthrough bleeding and need to be seen,'" she tells me, summoning authority and expertise in her voice. They scheduled her appointment. Six months after her first visit, she again saw Dr. Smith, who agreed her bleeding was a problem and increased her progestin dose in an effort to stabilize her cycles. This dose change worked, and Whitney was grateful for the reprieve after half a year of irregularity. I'm left frustrated while listening. This was the perfect opportunity to address her heavy bleeding *and* contraception together, yet in my mind, the doctor did not fully meet Whitney's needs.

Why do Black women have to self-diagnose their gynecologic problems? What about all of the women who would understandably toss out the progestin pills without ever knowing what was wrong? I asked Whitney why she didn't do just that. What made her keep seeking care despite a series of low-quality gynecologic interactions? She sighs and shrugs. "You just . . . you keep going," she tells me, echoing something she says she learned from her mother. "I wanted to figure it out." I recognize this characteristic in my friend from our work together. She doesn't leave data hanging, unexplained. She will get to the root of the matter, no matter how many questions it requires. It is why she is one of the best scientific collaborators I've worked with and, in this case, why she eventually got the contraception she needed at the appropriate dose for her body.

~

In most cases, heavy menstrual bleeding occurs when the uterine lining, or endometrium, sheds irregularly.† There are many treatments

---

* See chapter 3, "The Basics," for a helpful summary on the menstrual cycle phases.

† In chapter 9 of this book, I cover in detail how physicians diagnose heavy menstrual bleeding and its underlying causes. Because it is a symptom that can represent dozens of different conditions, we have a step-by-step approach to using both detailed patient diaries, imaging tests, and blood tests to narrow down and identify the ultimate cause. For now, we'll focus on the treatments for heavy menstrual bleeding.

that can be highly effective, including combined progesterone- and estrogen-containing pills, progesterone IUDs, and hormonal implants. However, too many Black individuals are mistrustful of these methods because of our community's history in medical contexts. It's not only our understanding of history that makes us skeptical. Many of us have ourselves experienced mistreatment in medical settings, especially in reproductive healthcare. Black women report, frequently, feeling coerced into accepting hormonal contraception—birth control—over their concerns and objections. This is a chilling echo of the type of reproductive control taken upon enslaved Black women compounded by the popularity of the stereotype that Black women are overly promiscuous and have too many children. It is a historical stereotype that is still undermining Black women's care. The legacy of harm has created a justified resistance in our community to hormonal treatments for bleeding.

I want to present heavy menstrual bleeding treatments here, without the oppressive context of a gynecologist's office and without the worry that this is all just about subversively pushing birth control. It is not. It is much more complex than that.

We can think about treatment for heavy menstrual bleeding in four buckets: stabilizing the endometrium, suppressing ovulation, destroying the endometrium, and removing the endometrium. We can build off the basics I shared in chapter 3 to understand how these different processes work.

Endometrial stabilization happens when we do something to increase the maturity of the endometrial tissue (which typically occurs during the secretory phase), make the blood vessels less leaky (those leaks typically occur during the menstrual phase), or both. Broadly speaking, there are three ways to do this, and usually it's a combination of approaches that will do the trick.

First, a common (but not universal) cause of endometrial destabilization is an excess of estrogen, the primary signal of the endometrium to grow. As mentioned in chapter 2, estrogen is secreted directly from ovarian cells but is also made in other areas of the body. There are several ways to adjust estrogen levels. Adipose (fat) cells make androgen, a hormonal precursor that is transformed into estrogen. This excess estrogen leads to overstimulation and overgrowth of the endometrium—causing irregular and heavy bleeding. In addition, regardless of fat cells, insulin—a hormone we produce in response to carbohydrate intake—impacts the menstrual cycle in two ways. First, insulin stimulates ovarian cells to produce androgens that are, as mentioned, transformed into estrogen. Second, insulin interrupts the brain signaling that triggers ovulation, resulting in inappropriately low progesterone levels. The result? Too much estrogen stimulation without the balancing progesterone. When any of these factors are driving abnormally heavy bleeding, then decreasing simple carbohydrate and sugar intake can improve the menstrual cycle—both in terms of regularity and amount of bleeding.* When there are fewer androgens from fat cells, there is less endometrial overgrowth from estrogen. When there are fewer insulin surges from sugar intake, or greater insulin regulation from exercise, there is endometrial overgrowth from estrogen. When the endometrium stops overgrowing, you get less irregular bleeding and lower overall bleeding during the menstrual cycle. The endometrium is stabilized by bringing estrogen levels back down to balance.

Second, the endometrium can also be stabilized by adjusting progesterone levels. Progesterone is a powerful signal that creates more structure in the endometrium and promotes maturation of the blood vessels, both of which mean that blood flow stays somewhat consistent during menstruation. Progesterone also activates those smooth muscle cells in the uterine lining that keep the vessels contracted so bleeding amounts are tightly regulated and you don't hemorrhage every month. You can stabilize the endometrium by increasing progesterone levels. Because increased progesterone blocks estrogen's effects, the top (superficial) endometrial layer eventually thins out over several months. You may continue to ovulate, but you do not have anything to shed. The bottom (basal) endometrial layer, the one with the stem cells that is critical for womb health and fertility, remains

* Exercise also decreases insulin levels, so committing to consistent physical activity may also improve heavy bleeding when high insulin is a driving cause. There is not as much data *in research* to confirm this cause and effect, but as we were taught in medical school, exercise is pretty much the "miracle drug."

happily quiet and intact.* Progesterone can be used alone, but often it is better paired with small amounts of estrogen to prevent "breakthrough bleeding," like the kind Whitney had. This allows the endometrium to adjust with a stable, constant level of this hormone.

Progesterone can be given to someone experiencing heavy menstrual bleeding in a number of ways. These include the following:

- Orally, with estrogen derivative in a pill or alone. (There is more breakthrough bleeding when it's used alone.)
- Vaginally, with a ring placed in the vagina where the progesterone is absorbed into the vaginal walls.
- In an intrauterine device (IUD), where a tiny amount of progesterone is released directly to the endometrium, and very little gets to the rest of the body. This is one of the most effective treatments of heavy menstrual bleeding.
- Through a patch (on top of the skin), a subdermal (under the skin) implant, or an injection.

A third way to stabilize the endometrium is with medications that alter the inflammatory cascade of menstruation.† As follows are two nonhormonal types of medications that do this:

- NSAIDs (examples: ibuprofen, naproxen sodium). These work because they decrease the prostaglandin proteins that kick off the endometrial breakdown in the menstrual cycle. You don't get as many leaky vessels, you get fewer inflammatory cells, and thus, less tissue breakdown and bleeding. We encourage folks to take them one to two days before a cycle starts, because be-

---

* The upper two-thirds of the endometrium is the superficial layer, which grows and sheds each month with a menstrual cycle. The basal layer does not grow and shed monthly but has a key role in providing the cells that regenerate the endometrium. For a full explanation of this, see the previous chapter 3 section on the endometrium.

† In chapter 3, I cover the menstrual cycle and how specifically the menstrual phase is made of up three steps: inflammation, hypoxia, and repair. The inflammatory step induces the breakdown of the endometrial tissue and its associated blood vessels.

fore you see blood, the inflammatory cascade (the *menstrual* phase) has already started. NSAIDs also help greatly with pain (see chapter 5).

- Tranexamic acid. This is a treatment that blocks the activation of a clot-busting enzyme (plasmin). The effect is that it preserves and bolsters early blood clots as they form in the endometrium, cutting off continued bleeding. It significantly cuts down on excessive bleeding because of this and is an important part of any effort to treat heavy menstrual bleeding.

Suppressing ovulation also treats heavy menstrual bleeding, as that stops the bleeding cycle altogether. It results in menstrual suppression. With no hormonal signals from the ovary, the endometrium doesn't enter the growth-and-shedding dance at all. Combination birth control pills, patches, and rings have this effect and so can be excellent treatments for heavy bleeding for those who can tolerate these interventions. *Combination* means they contain both an estrogen and progesterone and/or androgen-type hormone. Traditionally, these methods have been scheduled so that women still have a monthly (or quarterly) bleed by adding placebo pills for a week or advising removal of the patch or pill for a week. This simulates ovulation and prompts the endometrium to shed, but to a much smaller extent given the absence of true ovarian stimulation. For some women, this is an important ritual and that is fine. Having a simulated period is not biologically necessary, though. For many, the option of suppressing ovulation and therefore menstruation, essentially turning off your cycle, feels deeply unnatural. I understand this. In a world with increased artificiality everywhere, where the norm has become altering your appearance and biology in some way, shape, or form, I see women take to "natural cycles" as a way to claim authentic relationship to their bodies. There is nothing wrong with this, provided your cycles are, indeed, *normal*. It's also worth keeping in mind that before the invention of hormonal contraception, what was "natural" was to be pregnant a lot more often and thus have a lot *fewer* menstrual cycles over the course of a lifetime. If we are going to champion the rights of women and all folks with a uterus to a healthy sexual life without constantly being pregnant, we should acknowledge that we are actually cycling *much more* than we would be "naturally." I encourage us all not to frown upon methods to suppress ovulation and therefore menstruation, as 1) having fewer cycles more closely resembles the lifetime menstrual exposure of our ancestors, and 2) we must not believe we are meant to suffer. If endometrial stabilization methods are not enough to give someone back the quality of life they deserve, then menstrual suppression is safe, reasonable, and aligned with the experiences of our foremothers. Other stronger ovulation and menstrual suppression options are discussed in chapter 5, "Endometriosis."*

Endometrial destruction can stop heavy bleeding and periods, without impacting ovulation. We go back to the endometrial layers. The basal layer does not grow and shed monthly but has a key role in providing the stem cells that regenerate the endometrium. Destruction of this layer stops that process. Endometrial ablation is a procedure where the cervix is dilated and a camera is placed through it to see the endometrial lining in the uterine cavity. Ablation (burning and scarring of the lining) can then take place through different mechanisms—electricity, heat (heated fluid, radiofrequency, microwave), cold (cryoablation), or gas. All of these modalities destroy the superficial and deep (basal) endometrial layers. This can be an option for some people who don't want cycles, don't want hormones, and don't want reproductive capacity.

Endometrial removal. Finally, we have hysterectomy. There is a reason why hysterectomy is the second-most common surgery among women (after C-section). Hysterectomy rates have declined more than 40 percent since the 1990s and continue to drop. Still, approximately six hundred thousand such surgeries are performed in the United States each year. Removal of the uterus is definitive and provides many with an end to decades of suffering. It is also a surgery that is more than three times more common in young Black women

* Because I am a gynecologic oncologist and I hate cancer, I must also tell you that decreasing the "natural" number of ovulatory cycles significantly *decreases* the risk of ovarian cancer, which one in seventy women will get and is very deadly. This has been shown over and over again in decades of research—the less you ovulate, the lower your risk of ovarian cancer. Okay, back to the womb.

than their White peers. That's because the medical community is not discussing with Black women the less invasive, less permanent solutions discussed above, early enough. We will discuss hysterectomy many times in this book as a common end point to gynecologic suffering, welcomed by some and mourned by others. Whitney would welcome it, but not before a harrowing journey.

Whitney and Louis were married on April 14, 2013.* They were eager to have children, and Whitney soon got pregnant. Her first ultrasound showed she had a large, 7 cm fibroid in her uterine wall.† This did not worry my friend at all. She figured since she hadn't had any symptoms or problems with that fibroid up until now, there was nothing to worry about. "I think at that time I was just thinking about the pregnancy. To me, to have such a big fibroid and it hadn't been causing me any symptoms? I was just like, oh, okay, it's there," she recalls. "I didn't know as much about how things can change over the life course. . . . I think it just felt like if it hasn't bothered me now, it's probably not going to bother me later." She was receiving her pregnancy care at a birthing center with nurse midwives who felt the same. Though Whitney had some throbbing early on in pregnancy, for which she needed to take ibuprofen and rest, she was otherwise fine . . . until at twenty-two weeks pregnant when her bag of water broke (*ruptured membranes,* in obstetrics speak) far too early. She was at home, up late working on a research paper and formatting it just right to submit for publication. She felt liquid leave her body, and while that did strike her as odd, Whitney remained unconcerned. As she describes her disassociation in that moment, I can relate, given my own tendency to ignore troubling symptoms rather than imme-

* Their wedding was covered in *The New York Times,* a longtime dream of Whitney's. Vincent M. Mallozzi, "Whitney Robinson, Louie Rivers III," *New York Times*, April 14, 2014, https://www.nytimes.com/2013/04/14/fashion/weddings/whitney-robinson-louie-rivers-iii-weddings.html.

† A fibroid is a noncancerous smooth muscle tumor of the uterus; they are very common in Black women. I will go into great detail on these interesting players in chapter 6.

diately acknowledge them. Her plan was to submit the paper and go to bed. She would be practical and get her work done. It was Whitney's husband, Louis, who insisted they go in and get checked out at the birth center. The midwife on call confirmed that a major pregnancy complication had occurred. From there, the couple was quickly moved to the main university hospital, and about twenty-four hours later, I received the email my friend sent to our full research study team. Her message was filled with her usual professionalism and warmth and communicated that she was hospitalized indefinitely.

Whitney beat the odds and delivered a very healthy baby boy at thirty-four weeks. I remember being terrified for her during this time, but every time I went to visit during her weeks of bed rest, she was optimistic and calm. At the time, I wondered what kind of counseling she had received—and did she know the terrible odds? Now that we have been collaborators for over ten years, I understand more deeply her connection to science and data. She had looked into the research, saw the data and the poor odds of a healthy baby, and understood there was nothing for her to do but pray and stay calm. I wondered at the time if the fibroid was the issue. I asked her, and the answer was gray. Maybe, maybe not. The data grounded her, even though it didn't provide answers. The night before her induction was scheduled, she went into spontaneous labor and delivered by 6:00 the next morning.* She opted for a progesterone-containing IUD for birth control after delivery. She was thinking about contraception, but she received another big benefit. For the first time in her life, her periods were finally much lighter. "It was like a different world," she relates with eyes wide. It was great timing too. She had a baby to care for and her essential work in gynecology research to continue. She experienced several years of respite.

Whitney and Louis went on to have another healthy child four years later, this time with no complications. She again opted for the progesterone IUD after delivery. But after a few years, at the age of

* Of course, while approaching the goal she prayed for, thirty-four weeks of pregnancy, Whitney had read up on every single way to induce labor naturally and got going with it nonstop. It worked!

forty-two, something started to change. She recalls being out for her usual walk near her home one January day. My friend's eyes go distant as she tells me about the shift. "I was just out walking one day and I felt dizzy and disoriented. I even felt like it was a little bit dangerous to drive home . . . and it was just really weird." She was faint. She didn't have any energy and ended up in bed for twenty-four hours. She rested, hydrated, and got back to her routine. This would have been perhaps unremarkable as a single occurrence, but this went on to happen several times. Whitney thought she just needed to increase her daily water intake, which she did. She also wondered about perimenopause, so she started tracking all her symptoms to better understand what was happening. This insistence on data gathering, on being practical and looking at the facts, would create a detailed and disturbing account of the next two years of my friend's life. She generously shares her meticulous notes with me.

Date	Notes
Jan 15, 2022	*Bad dehydration (2); cramping?*
Jan 16, 2022	*Continued pain on each side of lower trunk / gut curve; late in day—feelings of constipation.*
Jan 17, 2022	*Filled a panty liner. More blood than usual.*

It's interesting to me that during our conversation she spoke mostly about dizziness and assumed dehydration, but her written account is clear on another symptom: a new increase in bleeding despite her having an IUD for several years. We live in a society that shuns all public discussions of periods, that makes little girls in a third-grade classroom who start to bleed feel they have to manage it all themselves. Collectively, we have such a low standard for gynecologic care that women call "good care" someone who at least talks to them. This silencing seeps into all of us. Even my friend, who grew up with a family wall calendar with *P*s and *WP*s in plain sight, still exhibited this powerful silencing in her retelling of her experience to me. Whitney was dizzy, she was fainting, she was having cramping (for the first time in her life), and she was *bleeding more and more* when she shouldn't have been.

This goes on and on. It's not until September of 2022 that she writes, "I hope this isn't gyn-related. Six ibuprofen pills helped a lot." Six. That's 1200 mg of ibuprofen after nine months of symptoms, increasing in pain and debilitation. In October, Whitney tried to wean herself off the ibuprofen but couldn't. She was using a heating pad daily, and she couldn't sleep. She was pulling out all the stops to manage her pain, and the bleeding continued.

Date	Notes
Sept 30, 2022	*I slept better (10:00 p.m.–12:00 a.m., 12:00–3:00 a.m., ragged after 3:00 a.m.) last night using the heating pad. I noticed blood in sheets and underwear around 6:00 a.m. today.* *** I Hope this isn't gyn-related.* *** 6 ibuprofen pills—helped a lot.*
Oct 2, 2022	*I tried to scale back on ibuprofen today: 2 pills—but I'm distractedly achy now at 9:00 p.m. despite heating pad at 8:15 p.m.; bowel pain starting again—not as sharp as first day but like that. ** I'll take 2 more pills.*

She had now started recording her bleeding days with red boxes in her tracker, rather than words. I see that in October, she bleeds for fifteen of the thirty-one days—essentially half. Yet Whitney was still attributing most of her pain as bowel-related.* By November, Whitney had developed heartburn (a classic consequence of heavy ibuprofen

* The uterus, bladder, and bowels all sit on top of one another in the pelvis, so this is completely understandable. In fact, doing careful exams and asking the right questions is exactly what gynecologists are trained to do to distinguish these things for people.

or NSAID use) and saw her PCP, whose visit note reads that she "reviewed potential causes of abdominal pain" with Whitney and "is reassured that her symptoms have improved." (I assume Whitney's pain would come and go, and perhaps that day, Whitney had begun to convince herself she was feeling better.) But Whitney continued to suffer.

It was now January 2023, one year after the start of her first concerning symptoms. Whitney had an idea: Maybe her IUD needed to be replaced. The birth center where she had received prenatal care had closed, and so she had to find new gynecologic care. She reached out to the nurse midwife who had diagnosed her ruptured membranes on that fateful night. On January 10, 2023, Whitney had an appointment with a colleague of that midwife, a gynecologist. That day, she had noted in her symptom tracker, *"Why am I bleeding so much?!"* (She had been bleeding for twelve days.) But when I review the notes from the appointment, I see no indication that Whitney was in a state of distress. Instead, the doctor simply notes that Whitney is a forty-two-year-old who has had two pregnancies and two births and who has come that day for an annual exam, including a Pap smear. The report includes a few lines about Whitney declining STI screening and the fact that she's completed the HPV vaccination series. And then it ends. "Follow up in 1 year for annual or [earlier] if needed."

This disconnect is profound. Whitney has spent a year suffering and needing intervention. Her gynecologist sees her as a standard patient there for an "annual exam"—which, by definition, is not problem-focused but rather a full assessment of health and well-being. The incorrect lens applied to Whitney is startling to me. She remembers being frustrated she couldn't get what she thought she went for that day, an IUD replacement. She remembers they explained that the IUD procedure had to be another visit, and they scheduled that follow-up appointment, a couple of months out. When Whitney showed up for that follow-up visit, there was yet another scheduling error, and they were again not set up to do IUD insertions that day. They rescheduled for months later, again.

By May 2023, Whitney was so limited in her activity that her daily tracker celebrated being able to do the smallest amount of movement: *"I felt okay at the beginning of the day. I even did a short walk and a 10-minute workout."* But mostly, the tracker chronicles her suffering, including a major unexpected event.

Date	Notes
May 26, 2023	*Weird liquidy peanut butter–colored discharge—sudden gush when watching Yellowjackets, episode 9.*
May 27, 2023	*In a lot of pain, stayed in bed most of day. Crampy, pain, some bowel pressure and nausea.*
May 31, 2023	*Felt okay at beginning of day. By midday bleeding escalated with a vengeance! Bled through pad and pants. Cramping pain is back as well. ** IUD expulsion!! ** Coughing still annoying and messed up sleep last night.*
June 1, 2023	*HUGE CLOTS TODAY, worse as day progressed, especially after I went out to [friend's] bday. Bled through pad, underwear, jeans, and dress.*
June 17, 2023	*SUDDEN gush of blood during morning exercise, including two big clots. A big shock!* 😳

In May, five months after she was seen by a gynecologist and seventeen months after her symptoms began, Whitney's body expelled her IUD. Even though the heavy bleeding continued after the IUD came out, she wondered if all her problems had been related to the contraceptive device.* She initially declined to get it replaced and hoped everything would get better and her symptoms would improve.

* People with large fibroids have an increased risk of expelling their IUD. It is not anywhere close to 100 percent, but if the pressure from the fibroids distorts the uterine cavity, it can be hard for the IUD to stay in place.

They didn't.

As I listen to Whitney, I wonder whether the clinicians she saw had considered the possible root causes of her symptoms. Had they reviewed all the possibilities, so they could run the tests, ask questions, and eventually discover the cause? She had pain and lightheadedness and fatigue and new bleeding out of nowhere. She had a 7 cm fibroid, and large fibroids are at risk of what we call *degeneration*. They can break down on their own, causing quite of bit of pain and inflammation and cramping. Where was the assessment of this fibroid?

In August of that same year, Whitney noticed a rash on her arm and googled to find out what it could be. Eczema? A sign of anemia? This prompted another PCP visit, where a blood test showed she was absolutely clinically anemic. Her red blood cell count, the final step 3 phase of iron deficiency, was too low. She was referred to a hematologist, who started her on iron transfusions. What did he think about the source of her anemia? "You should keep getting that gynecology stuff checked out," she remembers him telling her. She was shocked by how little consideration he gave to the most common cause of anemia in women. Meanwhile, she was also now having vulvar pain, increased pelvic pain, especially at bedtime, and the heavy bleeding that continued and remained unexplained.

Date	Notes
Aug 20, 2023	*I am bleeding SO much.*
Sept 9, 2023	*Intense exhaustion in evening. I did Peloton Matty's 10-minute low-impact aerobics. I couldn't get up from floor.*
Nov 29, 2023	*Worst cramping pain of my life!*

"I haven't communicated how disabled I was," Whitney tells me, referring to her documentation at the time. "I had a few good hours a day, you know. I was in bed by the afternoon, even when working from home," she detailed. "I would be on a call with my team and I just couldn't get through it. I really could barely work a half day at home, not going anywhere. I couldn't even sit up at the computer, past 2:00, 3:00 P.M." Despite having so little energy, mothering two kids under five years old, and *still working,* Whitney found the time to switch gynecologists. Realizing she hadn't gotten better by avoiding a new IUD, and remembering her initial relief with her first IUD, she tried a repeat IUD insertion in September of 2023. But it was to no avail. She had an ultrasound that was interpreted as normal, other than her known fibroid.

By October 2023, nearly two years after her first fainting spell, Whitney was done. Her pain was no longer eased by ibuprofen. This late in her journey, she was given a few types of endometrial stabilization medications, norethindrone and tranexamic acid, for a few weeks without success. My friend was ready for a hysterectomy. She found a surgeon who would do one. She still had to wait several months for a surgery date. In December 2023, her log notes, *"A lot of bleeding: Super tampon and huge overnight pad just to make it a couple hours. Still spillover."* She canceled a much-anticipated family trip home because she could not imagine traveling in her condition.

Whitney had a hysterectomy on February 19, 2024. Her official diagnosis and indication for surgery was *chronic pelvic pain and abnormal uterine bleeding from a fibroid.* Her surgical findings included a uterus that was stuck to her anterior abdominal wall with thick, dense adhesions, an appendix fused to the back of her uterus, a degenerating fibroid, and pus-filled fluid in her pelvis. Forty percent of her uterine wall was taken up by degenerating fibroid tissue. Whitney had a severe infection in her uterus, a uterine wall filled with calcified degenerating fibroids, and an appendix that had tunneled into her uterine wall, aflame with infection. She had a multi-organ infection that had gone completely undiagnosed.

The medical notes Whitney has gathered from her official record do not make sense when read alongside the personal journal she kept. In fact, the two sets of documents reveal a jarring disconnect between her suffering and what was perceived. Whitney must have brought up the possibility of infection during medical appointments, as I noticed that there are at least two entries where the notes indicate reassurance. She was told that "if you had an infection, you would be feeling quite ill." My friend was so debilitated that she could barely make it through a few hours of work while sitting down at a computer. She had not slept well in *two years*.

"I tried to get good care, but I don't think I got great care. I think it's just so impossible. Like, how are people supposed to get good care?" Whitney and I sit with that question for a while, in silence.

She thinks about how she was both seen and not seen. At clinical visits, she was always asked to rate her pain: How severe was it, on a scale of 0 to 10? She would say 8.

Whitney continues, "But then my surgeon afterward, she's like, 'You must have been in so much pain.' Like, she really seemed shocked." I am at a loss for words as Whitney processes this out loud with me. "I thought to myself, 'I told you I was an eight.' I didn't actually say out loud to her again, but I realized then that there was a disconnect." She continues, "Like, I was trying so hard to give an accurate assessment. . . . [But] are they going to think I'm hysterical if I say too much? And then also there's all this self-managing about how I present. I think it backfired on me."

Whitney goes on to share that she was simply too capable. There were other people in her life who didn't realize she was that sick, including me, and I feel guilty about that in retrospect. She said that she would schedule her medical appointments in the morning because she knew her energy would be gone by the afternoon. She didn't look as sick to her doctors because they weren't seeing her at her worst time of day. She sums up a perspective I completely understand: "I wanted to present the best version of myself to care as opposed to 'see me at my worst, caretakers, and help me.'"

I'm struck hard by this. My friend was so debilitated she couldn't make it past three hours of activity in the morning. So, she scheduled all her doctor visits early in the day because she couldn't even make it out of the house later. Not being able to make it to the outpatient clinic due to debilitation is typically grounds for hospital admission. It speaks to a problem so severe that urgent intervention is needed.

Whitney is a decorated, brilliant epidemiologist. And a Black woman. To the healthcare system, her suffering was invisible. The strength and practicality she was raised with, the strength and practicality required of her as a smart Black woman in a world that can't see her as vulnerable, masked her suffering.

While pulling out all stops to try to help herself, Whitney was also working with me on a significant and related professional undertaking. Since 2016, we had been building a dataset from thousands of healthcare records across the state of North Carolina to create a symptom severity index for gynecologic conditions. This was Whitney's flagship research project, designed to understand why Black women had higher hysterectomy rates in the Deep South. Was it the severity of their symptoms or overtreatment by uncaring doctors? We needed a way to objectively compare symptoms using the medical records—and there wasn't one. We did the work to design it. Whitney and I were having sometimes weekly research meetings about symptoms like heavy bleeding, periods lasting longer than seven days, pelvic pressure resulting in incontinence, and how many gynecology visits about one problem should qualify as *severe*. This is what we talked about all of the time for five years, yet I had no idea that she was living this nightmare. I share this reflection with Whitney, aware that we have both shed tears during our conversation and that my words may bring about more. Whitney shares with me that her career coach at the time also noticed this disconnection between her private suffering and the topics of her professional research. She had suggested that Whitney apply our newly developed symptom severity scale to herself and assess where she would fall. Whitney never did. Why?

"Some of it's like . . . then what do I do with that information?" she said when I asked her. "Maybe I was compartmentalizing, and I wanted to keep compartmentalizing because I want to keep thinking I can overcome this. And maybe seeing that like, oh, *I'm* that severe patient. Maybe that would've felt overwhelming and stopped me in my tracks in a way that I didn't want to acknowledge. And I think I still felt like, well, this is bad, but there are so many more people who are suffering more than me. . . . I think I still was minimizing."

Whitney told me the inequity in our systems make her sick to her stomach. Even as she was frustrated by how long she had to wait for surgery, she knew there were people waiting many months longer. As hard as it was for her to get a gynecologist to listen, she ultimately was able to do so. "I think it is overwhelming to me to then realize the depth of what other people are experiencing."

Her words make me think of her bleeding on towels in bed as a little girl. I'm filled with empathy at how early she learned to take care of severe symptoms in her life, and how deeply ingrained suffering would be when your threshold of "normal" is set at such a young age. I think about how our gynecology systems would leave it to her to deem her bleeding was "too much" before we, as trained healthcare providers, would deem it so. Why would we abdicate our responsibility to minimize suffering for something so important when we know women, and especially Black women and all those with a uterus, suffer so much?

With the benefit of her personal journal and tracking data paired with her medical records, here's what I think happened with Whitney: She had a large 7 cm fibroid that started to degenerate (break down and die). When fibroids start dying, an inflammatory reaction occurs that can create changes in the menstrual cycle and off-cycle bleeding. She felt lightheaded and tired, was dehydrated, and had bleeding changes. Eventually, her IUD was expelled from her body due to all this disordered bleeding and inflammation. And then—a reminder here that I am *guessing* using the benefit of my years as a clinician and researcher—a new IUD was inserted (after her original was expelled) into an already fragile, inflamed uterus, and an infection took hold. It's not clear to me whether this was caused by poor sterile technique, or if she was already vulnerable to an infection after months and months of inflammation, or both. Either way, her lab records show that her white blood cell count, a marker of infection, increased after the insertion—something Whitney points out to me as well. She had more pain, more cramping, and more bleeding as her uterus desperately tried to clear itself. After two years of suffering, it makes all the sense in the world to me that Whitney would essentially demand a hysterectomy. And I have to wonder what her path would have looked like if any of her gynecologic concerns—her fibroid, her heavy bleeding throughout her entire life, her increased cramping, her ongoing, continuous, severe debilitation—had been taken seriously immediately and evaluated fully.

Whitney's gynecology story is just one of several difficult accounts in her family. She told me about her aunt, a "superstrong woman" who as a girl would stay home every month from severe pain with periods. This is a characteristic highly suggestive of endometriosis. As soon as she got to college, this aunt sought out birth control. This hadn't been an option before leaving home, as the aunt was not allowed to have what Whitney's grandmother only saw as a contraceptive medication and not a treatment to relieve suffering. Whitney's mother had bad bleeding and likely fibroids when Whitney was a teenager, and had a hysterectomy in her forties. Whitney jokes about how her mother changed a lot after that and perhaps some of her mother's less attractive personality traits were just the result of a woman suffering in silence. Whitney's grandmother died of uterine cancer.

These stories cover the range of gynecologic conditions that disproportionately affect Black women. Having covered heavy menstrual bleeding here, we'll dive into the rest of the conditions in subsequent chapters. They are stories of suffering, silencing, and neglect. If you are thinking that Whitney's story seems complicated, it is. My goal is to break down these conditions one by one. I offer you a clearer understanding of each condition so you can see how they may work together to create confusion and suffering and sometimes even death.

CHAPTER 5

ENDOMETRIOSIS

The Painful Womb

When I was unable to become pregnant after cycle tracking and timed intercourse for eight months, I sought medical advice. The battery of tests I went through came back normal, and I was given a diagnosis of "unexplained infertility." I was shaken and especially disappointed in the White face of infertility support and care, where I had no options to see a Black specialist despite living in a Southern state where a full quarter of the population was Black. Not to mention the websites and support groups that didn't feature anyone who looked like me. I was embarrassed and lonely, yet still had to hold up my mask of competence as the only Black woman in the room. Though the journey was one I would not wish on anyone, we eventually succeeded after multiple rounds of IVF treatments. When I delivered three weeks early by C-section, the doctors told me I had severe scarring on my uterus, fallopian tubes, and ovaries: classic signs of endometriosis.

I thought back to my childhood and my horribly painful periods. Every month, like clockwork, I suffered. When I received the diagnosis of endometriosis, soon after giving birth to my first child, I wondered: How had I, an ob-gyn

in training, lived through that amount of monthly pain, and pain between cycles, without ever considering that I might need a diagnosis?

Given the impact endometriosis has on women's lives, it is shameful how little we know, how few effective treatments there are, and how comparatively late in life we come to understand that we even have the condition. Unfortunately, my experience of receiving a diagnosis due to my desire to become a mother is common. We often narrow the public discourse and many private doctor-patient medical conversations on endometriosis to one simple question: Can you get pregnant? But endometriosis affects nearly every single body system, not just the reproductive system. It twists organs beyond repair and causes a fire of inflammation in the pelvis that can feel like we are walking around with broken glass inside of us. That is why the main sign of endometriosis is pain. Someone living with the condition typically experiences outsize pain with periods and continued pain between cycles.

The term *endometriosis* was coined by Dr. John Sampson in the 1920s as part of a growing interest in the problem of infertility among White middle- and upper-class women. At the time—and some might argue the same is true today—the ability of these women to reproduce was considered of paramount importance. The central value of women was to ensure the continued population of this ruling class in society. Miscegenation laws made cross-racial marriage and, by proxy, procreation, illegal. Doctors noticed that endometriosis was more common among career-oriented women, particularly those who had decided to delay childbearing. This led to the biomedical community's classification of endometriosis as a "lifestyle" disease caused by these women's choices to face the stressors associated with working instead of being a homemaker, their more natural state in the patriarchal imagination.* They followed a long-repeated script of

* Right now, in 2025, the so-called tradwife aesthetic and movement is growing on social media and is a distressingly common talking point from the US executive branch of the government. The more this dangerous perspective is mainstreamed,

blaming women for any conditions that they did not biologically understand. Studies of endometriosis during this time organized patients into three groups: White women in private hospital wards, less-well-off White women in public wards, and all Negro women. Early medical literature proclaimed that Black women were less civilized and therefore not subject to the stress of modern life. As such, endometriosis had to be rare to nonexistent in this group. Another prominent figure in gynecologic history, Dr. Joseph Meigs, was fond of contrasting the infertility of civilized White women to the rampant fertility of monkeys. The White women were worthy of empathy and investigation; the monkeys were not. I can't see this gross choice of using fertile monkeys as the metaphorical opposite to infertile White women outside of the long history of comparing Black people to animals, and especially monkeys. The unstated message is clear to me: Black women were uncivilized, naturally fertile, and easily conceptualized as animals.

In a 1976 article in the *American Journal of Obstetrics & Gynecology,* Dr. Donald L. Chatman, an African American gynecologist in Chicago, Illinois, noted that Dr. Meigs's theories conflicted with the reality he saw every day with the Black patients he cared for in his private practice. He collected data on nearly two hundred Black women who needed surgery and noted that in a full 20 percent of them, he found evidence of endometriosis in their bodies. Even more disturbingly, nearly 40 percent of these patients had been misdiagnosed with pelvic inflammatory disease. Pelvic inflammatory disease (PID) is a consequence of untreated sexually transmitted diseases that move from the vagina and cervix to infect the uterus, tubes, ovaries, and pelvis. Black women living under the shadow of ever-present racial promiscuity stereotypes had sought care with Dr. Chatman anyway, because of the extent of their pain and suffering. Prior to meeting him, they had not been met with empathy and investigative curiosity but with sexualized assumptions and disregard. Although Dr. Chatman and others challenged Drs. Sampson's and Meig's harm-

the more womb conditions will go back to being "lifestyle" diseases that are our fault and not worthy of care. All women must beware.

ful and incorrect ideas about race, class, and endometriosis, the latter's voices held sway for decades.

In the 1980s, there was finally an explicit shift away from these racist theories into a broader view of endometriosis from an environmental and genetic perspective. Larger studies were launched and new theories investigated, but Black women were still too often excluded from the research. Today, Black women living with this condition still face racial profiling, silencing, and delayed care.

This erasure is particularly devastating, because the risk factors of endometriosis are more common among Black girls and women. Most diseases don't start when we notice them. They start much earlier during critical windows of exposure and development when our cells are most malleable and cellular changes can have long-term consequences. For endometriosis, three of the five strongest risk factors during these early critical windows are known to be more common among Black individuals: being small for gestational age while in fetal development; having low birth weight at the time of birth; and having their first period at an early age. In fact, the earlier a person starts their periods, and the longer and heavier those periods are, the higher the chance is that they develop endometriosis. When all the risk factors are more common in a group, it follows that the condition is more common in that group too.

Black and White women have the same rate of endometriosis, according to studies that rely on hospitalization data or surgical pathology results. But this research is limited to who is able to navigate the myriad barriers to entry to get through the hospital door. To do so means the person living with the condition has recognized their pain as real and abnormal, can access a trained gynecologic specialist, can convince that doctor their pain is worth the investigative effort, and is financially, socially, and emotionally able to undergo the surgery necessary to receive the correct diagnosis. In our society, the odds are against Black women at every turn of this process.

This was certainly the case for Mya, a colleague of mine with whom I reconnected in 2024 at an international cancer research conference in San Diego that drew twenty-three thousand scientists eager to delve into the latest developments in their field. As a cancer epidemiologist, Mya Roberson, PhD, was one of them.

Mya is in her mid-thirties, lives with endometriosis, and graciously agreed to speak to me about her gynecologic memories and all facets of her life they touch. On the day we meet in my hotel room, she is the picture of composure. She wears an emerald-green dress and a stylish pink blazer, and her natural curls defy gravity and effortlessly pop with bounce and definition. She sits with her legs crossed at the ankles, her hands clasped in her lap, perfectly poised. Mya is a light-skinned Black woman, with a White mother and a Black father. As we begin, I'm curious about how my thoughts about Black mothers, daughters, and the womb will intersect with Mya's experience.

Mya grew up in rural Pennsylvania and was close to her mother, who worked in small-town family-owned diners frequented by working-class patrons throughout Mya's life. As a child, Mya spent many hours sitting at one of the empty restaurant tables playing Pokémon, doing her homework, or daydreaming about her future while her mother finished her shifts. She remarks on how much time they got to spend together despite how hard her mother worked and how limited their means were. "No dream was ever too big for me. The sky was my limit always," Mya says as she wistfully recalls her mother in those days. "She truly believed I could do absolutely anything I dreamed of and I deserved the world."

When Mya was nine, she bled through her pajamas while at a friend's house for a sleepover. She was surprised, but not shocked. Her mother had told her, in somewhat vague terms, that her body would be changing and one of the things that would happen was this kind of bleeding. But she was surprised to have it happen so soon, before she even hit her double digits.

The night she started bleeding, Mya's mother came to pick her up and gave her a more detailed talk about periods. Mya learned she would now get them every month, for a long time, and how to manage them with pads and tampons. Though Mya confesses she couldn't quite grasp the implications of bleeding "for the indefinite future," she felt calmed and comforted by her mother's instructions.

"She told me this was normal, that she too had started her cycles younger than her friends, and so we were the same in that." Mya took on this new responsibility well. She learned how to estimate time between bathroom trips at school and determine whether she could partake in the recess game based on what day her cycle was. She also felt a new distance between herself and her schoolmates. "I didn't have words for it at the time, but I think now what I was feeling was resentment," she told me. "They could go on playing and didn't have to worry like I did. I grew up in a rural small town; we didn't have any kind of sex ed until I was twelve. So, I think I was resentful that I had to deal with this and they didn't. I had to miss pool trips in the summer and say no to sleepovers." Mya would share her reasons for not going with a few friends, but mostly she never gave explanations.

There was something else she noticed about her newfound status as a girl who got periods. She was met with suspicion. The onset of puberty was one more thing that set her apart as the only Black girl in her school and often the only Black girl in any social setting in town. "I found this kind of judgment. Other kids' parents were wondering why I knew all of these things that I knew so young. They would look at me and my mom [suspiciously]." Mya learned to keep quiet, to keep being a bright, academically gifted third-grade student, and to keep dreaming.

To explain endometriosis, there are three primary theories* for why endometrial-like tissue shows up where we don't expect it. The first is that it gets lost. In the shedding (menstrual) phase of the cycle, where this tissue is supposed to head down and out of the womb, it

* These theories (and more) are constantly under debate and refinement, at the time of writing this chapter. The scientific conversation is less about them not being true, but more about how complicated and perhaps intertwined they are as they each explain different aspects of the disease, but no one theory explains everything. I respect these nuances and strive in these pages to create a simple view of how the body can operate, so everyone can appreciate how endometriosis may work in the body.

makes a wrong turn and flows backward. Instead of moving down and out the front door—the vagina—it moves up and through the fallopian tubes, the back door, where the end destination is not a tampon, a pad, or on a bad day, your favorite sweatpants. Instead, the end destination is deeper into your body—namely, your pelvis and abdominal cavity. It's in the wrong place, but it's still in the body. It's not the right environment, it's not the womb, but this tissue adapts. It takes root in these new spaces and keeps doing its job, growing and shedding.

The second cause for endometriosis is a bit more magical, for lack of a better word. Whether this happens spontaneously or because of the migrated endometrial-like cells that have shown up to wreak a little havoc, we are not sure. What we do know is that the *peritoneum* tissue that coats the inside of the pelvis can transform into endometrial-like tissue. This transformed tissue starts to release hormones. It starts to respond to hormones just as endometrial tissue does, and now you've got womb tissue where it should not be, making friends with the lost cells that have come to stay.

The third way endometriosis comes to be is the least common, but to me the most impressive in that it involves what I can't help but imagine as a deliberate, risky, big leap. Endometrial-like cells that have only ever been in the womb jump into either the blood vessels or the lymph system, the fast-moving highways of our bodies. They ride this whole-body system to worlds completely unknown. This is how endometriosis ends up in the lungs, the adrenal glands, or the belly button. These cells have jumped into a portal and are then sloshed around the body and deposited randomly in unknown territory. And they *survive*. This is likely why the earlier your cycles start and the heavier and longer your periods are, the higher the risk of endometriosis. The more "menstrual exposure" you have, the more chances you have for the endometrium to act up, get lost, recruit some nosy neighbors, and jump ship entirely to parts unknown.

I see endometriosis as a story of migration, transformation, appropriation, and maladaptation. As the womb cells move around the body, their survival is prioritized at the expense of the larger organism (us!). Our best guess is that genetic (inherited) and epigenetic (changes to how our DNA is expressed that we can be born with or acquire during our lifetime) factors drive this maladaptation of endometriotic tissue. Since we are not born inherently programmed with all these changes, we assume they likely come from our environment, whether that is at the macro level (e.g., from elements of our neighborhood, environmental toxins, food supply, etc.) or the micro level (e.g., from our chronic stress levels, sleep habits, etc.).* Or perhaps these changes come about randomly. I know we hate that explanation, but some things are in fact random. Our cellular processes—that turn DNA into RNA and then RNA into proteins—are riddled with places where errors can happen. We call these *somatic* mutations, and they happen all the time.†

Whatever the reason behind their unexpected behavior, the endometriotic cells do not act alone. To achieve each of these migratory feats and transformations requires an interaction of the endocrine (hormonal), inflammatory, immune, vascular, genetic, and nervous systems. These pathways are all involved, which is why treating and preventing endometriosis is not simple. It's not as simple as removing soy from your diet or avoiding handstands while on your period.

It's also not as simple as recognizing and communicating symptoms that are then easily understood by clinicians. Because endometriosis also changes your brain. These migrated lesions adapt and survive in their new environment while retaining their ability to grow, shed, and bleed. They also learn how to foster the growth of new *sensory nerve cells*. These nerve cells, which detect painful stimuli, were not there before and normally would not be there at all. We have many more nerve cells on the outside of our bodies (i.e., on our skin) than on our internal organs. These new sensory nerve cells create new sensitive neural pathways to the brain, which results in the brain's

* Very recently, endometriosis has been linked to autoimmune conditions such as rheumatoid arthritis, celiac disease, and psoriasis and may share some common genetic correlations. This research may open up more cross-treatment options for these conditions, as well as give more insight into how they come to be. Stay tuned.

† Endometriosis has even been reported (very, very, very rarely) in those assigned male at birth and folks born without a uterus. The human body contains what we call *pluripotent* cells that can transform into . . . anything. Wild.

increased ability to feel what's happening at that endometriosis location. When the newly sensitive place is the site of inflammation and bleeding, it *hurts*. This happens day in and day out, year in and year out. Most people with endometriosis wait years to be diagnosed. And while waiting, we experience chronic pain that changes us in fundamental ways.

It's hard for Mya to pinpoint when pain with her periods entered her life. "I can't remember when it wasn't there," she tells me. "I think from the beginning." It was just part of the experience, another reason to stay home and avoid activities when the bleeding began. In high school, Mya was a powerful discus thrower and shot-putter on her high school's track-and-field team. Just like the colleague I have come to know and respect deeply, Mya was a team player back then too. But when her cycles came, her pain became so bad she could barely compete. She remembers being laid out on the benches in the team locker rooms struggling to get up and get into uniform. "I wanted to be out there and I didn't want to let them down. But also, I couldn't move. It really hurt." Still, she never missed a track meet despite the pain. "I powered through," she remembers.

Mya, like many teen girls then, loved paging through *Teen Vogue, Elle Girl,* and similar youth-oriented magazines. She remembers coming across an article about birth control, specifically how it could be used to make your periods less painful. She felt some hope and immediately took it to her mother, whose response was loving, well-intentioned . . . and wrong. She told Mya it wasn't time for her to be thinking about birth control and she was skeptical about its effectiveness for period pain. Her own periods were painful and Mya would be okay, she said. And so, the girl pushed through.

Mya was the first person in her family to go to college, and she earned admission to Brown, an Ivy League school, in the fall of 2012. It was there, away from home for the first time and now sexually active, that Mya decided to try to seek help. She noticed how much more painful her periods seemed to be than her friends'. Although used to being an outsider in her small town, while living there, she hadn't connected that her painful periods were also far outside of normal. Now she was sure her cycles were too much. She was in pain, bedridden, and avoiding social activities every month, much more so than her friends. A new symptom had also come on board: painful sex. "I knew this was the time I was supposed to be having fun in school, learning about myself and relationships, including sex, and it just felt like this barrier," she tells me, excitement in her voice. "I just knew it could be better, that there was a way that I didn't have to be in so much pain."

I am intrigued because her mother, whom she trusted and respected, had essentially told her that her pain was normal. Why did Mya believe that she had options beyond the pain? I asked. Mya wasn't sure herself, but I chalk it up to the strength of a Black girl's dreaming, the same strength her mother seemed to have deliberately nurtured in her, recognizing her status as an outsider in their small town. It worked. Mya could reach for the sky and was worthy of achieving any dream she had, even the ones her mother couldn't see.

Mya went to campus health services and saw a doctor. She detailed her symptoms—painful periods, painful sex—and asked for help. Her doctor's presumptive diagnosis? Pelvic inflammatory disease (PID) related to an untreated sexually transmitted infection. One hundred years after the misogynist, racist medical rhetoric published by Sampson and Meigs, and nearly forty years after the good Dr. Chatman tried to correct the record, Mya was met with the same assumption—a Black woman with pelvic pain had to have PID. Mya's face is somehow both deadpan and confused as she looks at me, recounting this. "It didn't make sense. I went home and looked it up. I didn't have any of the risk factors. I only had ever had one sexual partner. I didn't have any symptoms like fever or anything. It didn't sound like me at all." PID causes pelvic pain but also symptoms of infection, such as fever, an elevated white blood cell count, and fatigue. Mya had none of those. Not only that, her cervical swab for any STIs came back negative. In a follow-up visit, despite the negative test, the campus doctor told her that she still felt Mya had PID, that sometimes the "swabs could be wrong." "I don't know how many swabs I got that year," she tells me. "They were all negative, and I was still in so much pain."

Mya took it upon herself to do more research. She knew she didn't have PID, but she still didn't know what she actually did have. After reading through medical articles, she came up with her own diagnosis: endometriosis. She went back to the campus doctor and reported her findings. "She just looked at me, and after a pause, she said, 'You know, I think you may be right.'" After a year and a half of chasing after phantom PID, the doctor wrote Mya a referral to see an off-campus gynecologist, as now she had a condition that was beyond the bounds of management of campus health.

Mya followed up quickly, eager to get real treatment for her real condition. She pauses before she continues, apparently preparing to relay this next anecdote as she shifts on the couch. "This is one of my most salient memories," she says. "I will never forget this." Mya was referred to an older White male gynecologist. She recounted her story to him, repeating details she had shared with her previous doctor. He examined her, and then he offered his expert opinion. "Yes, I agree that you likely do have endometriosis. But, right now, I want you to just focus on graduating college." Mya was a junior. He had just confirmed her diagnostic suspicions. She likely did have a debilitating chronic condition that causes immense pain, impacts multiple other organ systems, and can lead to infertility. And his prescription? Focus on your schoolwork. Mya, who was twenty at the time, left and continued to do what she had been doing for over a decade. She pushed through.

It is estimated that about 10 percent, or one in ten, of reproductive-age individuals with a uterus have endometriosis. Each endometriosis case costs over $10,000 per person diagnosed. This is on par with costs related to a single case of diabetes or rheumatoid arthritis, common conditions that don't bear the stigma of women's health. But unlike diabetes, RA, thyroid conditions, or anemia, endometriosis cannot be found on a blood test. In many cases, it can't even be found on our most common imaging tool for the pelvis, an ultrasound.*

Endometriosis is diagnosed primarily through direct surgical visualization. Someone must look inside our bodies to see whether the telltale lesions exist. When a diagnosis is so difficult to pin down that one needs surgery to verify it, there are many barriers to confirmation. As a result, endometriosis is grossly underdiagnosed. A review of over one hundred endometriosis studies estimated that up to 21 percent of women hospitalized for pelvic pain have endometriosis. Think about that for a moment. Of women who have pain severe enough to go to the hospital, one in five have endometriosis. This means the actual number of women with endometriosis is likely much higher, as many women suffer on their own, experiment with home remedies, and continue meeting their work, school, and caregiving responsibilities because they feel they have no other choice but to keep pushing through the pain. Those women go uncounted. Black women are more likely to be these women, taught to prioritize others first, taught to be excellent in the face of racism and sexism, and taught—ultimately—that we manage our own pain.

Diagnosing endometriosis is the perfect storm of what we call *nonspecific* symptoms. These are signals of the body's distress that could come from many different sources and thus are not specific to just one diagnosis. We also lack a reliable blood test that could help distinguish endometriosis from other things. Sometimes imaging can help. For example, if endometriosis is in the ovary, it can show up as a mass on an ultrasound or CT scan or MRI. If there are very deep lesions that are thick and extensive, we can see that on MRI. But many lesions are on

* Routine pelvic ultrasounds often miss endometriosis because some of the subtler signs that can visualize scarring and adhesions take special training to detect. So, endometriosis is often not seen on ultrasound and women are told that "everything looks normal." While progress in preoperative imaging with dynamic ultrasound has been made over the past several years, these techniques are not widely utilized, especially in the United States.

the surface of the body's interior tissue (*peritoneum*) and are not big and so are not picked up by these tools.*

And that is why surgery remains the gold standard diagnostic tool. The approach typically used is a laparoscopy, which involves using a small camera that usually enters the flesh at or above the belly button so a doctor can see for herself what's going on in a patient's pelvis and abdomen. Surgeons tend to minimize the apprehension patients have around surgery, because we do it every day. To me, a laparoscopy is minor compared to taking out a watermelon-size uterus, doing the complex work of removing cancers from a patient's bowels, or carefully dissecting out the sensitive ureters deep in the pelvis that hug your body's major blood vessels. But I do recognize that anytime someone is being put to sleep, completely under the control of other humans, and the body is being entered and viewed, it *is* a big deal. There are risks to any surgery, no matter how small.

The challenge for my colleagues and me is to be discerning about rushing someone to this diagnostic operation while also making sure we are not delaying or denying care. Women see an average of four doctors before being diagnosed correctly with endometriosis. That statistic is based on White women, so you can imagine how Black women fare in their search for an accurate diagnosis. When all you have is reporting your symptoms (painful periods, painful bowel movements, painful sex) and imaging tests that only pick up some lesions, you are highly dependent on the privilege of having a well-trained, empathetic gynecologist who will listen to you, believe you, and is capable of completing your surgery. The nation's disinvestment in women's health and gynecologic conditions and surgeons, in particular, makes this a difficult journey. Mya was living this nightmare.

---

* Some clinical settings with special expertise in imaging can detect endometriosis by ultrasound, but this requires the endometriosis to have *already caused* some subtle anatomic changes like inflammation that sticks the uterus to the ovary or pulls the rectum up higher than it should be. For ultrasound to detect the endometriosis, it already needs to have changed normal anatomy.

Mya left that hard-won but ultimately useless gynecology appointment disappointed, but like any of her goals, she did not give up on her dream of getting help for her painful periods. By this time, her bowel movements had also become painful, especially around the time of her cycles. She went back to "good old Google," as she calls it, did more research on endometriosis, and learned about surgical treatments. She became determined to find a new type of specialist she had recently learned of: a minimally invasive gynecologic surgeon, or MIGS. She learned how to identify them by looking for the acronym and additional evidence of fellowship training. With no hope of receiving quality care in Rhode Island, she focused on finding someone close to her childhood home so she could schedule an appointment during a break from school.

She found one. Dr. Karen Taverna-Miller was a MIGS-trained, full-service ob-gyn. Mya saw her during the fall break of her senior year and laid out the specifics of her situation again. This time, she was in the company of an expert who heard her. "She was clear, she believed me, and she had a plan," Mya said, *glowing* as she spoke of Dr. Taverna-Miller. "I was so relieved." They planned for Mya to have a diagnostic laparoscopy. Then, if Dr. Taverna-Miller found endometriosis, she had Mya's permission to safely remove as much of it as she could. Mya's mother was at her side while she awaited surgery and when she woke up. At Mya's postoperative visit, Dr. Taverna-Miller patiently went through her findings at surgery, showing Mya pictures and using drawings to explain her condition.

Mya did in fact have endometriosis, and it was extensive. Most notably, it had gone so far as to fuse her colon with her anterior body wall, which explained Mya's painful bowel movements and her pain with deep penetration during intercourse. "It all made sense, finally." Dr. Taverna-Miller had been able to remove most of the endometriosis lesions she found in Mya's pelvis, but not all of them. "Some of them were too risky because they were deeply infiltrating and had a higher risk of bleeding. She explained to me that I would need to take a hormonal suppression medication—Lupron—after surgery to help get rid of those pharmacologically." Dr. Taverna-Miller was clear to Mya that six months on the hormonal medication would make her feel worse before she felt better but that long term it would help her. Mya was fully on board and completed that course, though it was very challenging. "It was rough, I'm not going to lie. The mood swings were intense." Mya became depressed on the medication and even had moments of suicidal ideation. "But I remember thinking that I knew why I was doing it, and I really trusted her that she was fighting this thing along with me."

How did Mya feel afterward? "Like a whole new person. It was amazing. I could have sex without pain. I didn't have to stay in the house and avoid activities on my period. It was so good." I am happy for her even though I know there is much more to her journey.

As Mya's story shows, there are treatments for endometriosis. I want to scream this from the rooftops. There are treatments for endometriosis! They are not perfect, because nothing is. They don't work in every single person, because nothing does. But they help a lot of women a great deal, and I want Black women to be aware of and fully empowered to request and demand, if necessary, these treatments because we will no longer tolerate the "suffering as natural" narrative.

PHARMACOLOGICAL TREATMENT OF ENDOMETRIOSIS

Often, especially when a patient's lesions are less extensive than Mya's were, a gynecologist will begin with prescribing a medication to resolve the endometriosis lesions. The endometrium is a hormonally sensitive tissue. Migrated endometrial-like tissue can also adapt to release additional hormones and fuel its own growth. For these reasons, hormones are a big part of endometriosis treatment. We meet fire with fire. But let's get a lot more specific.

Estrogen is the hormone that promotes endometrial growth. So, to inhibit the growth of these migrated tissues, you need to either 1) *decrease* estrogen levels, 2) change the *impact* estrogen has on the endometriosis tissue, or 3) both. Low-fat, high-fiber diets are associated with lower levels of estrogen in the bloodstream. It follows that these diets would help decrease endometriosis symptoms, but currently there is not direct evidence for diet alone as an effective endometriosis treatment.* Medications that decrease estrogen levels and tend to be tolerated well by patients include estrogen-progesterone combination pills, patches, or rings. The progesterone decreases estrogen, and the estrogen provides what the body needs without introducing so much that it triggers endometrial growth.

Progesterone-only medications can also work, but they often have side effects people don't like, such as irregular spotting, headaches, and weight gain. Stronger medications, such as Lupron, a GnRH (gonadotropin releasing hormone) antagonist, suppress the body's estrogen-producing impulse entirely. Because these work hard to suppress estrogen, someone taking this type of medication will need to take low-dose estrogen to prevent menopause-like symptoms. Newer medications that work similarly, like elagolix and relugolix, come in oral formulations with some hormonal elements added back so they have fewer side effects and can be taken for longer. These are particularly promising, as they improve moderate and severe endometriosis symptoms and can be taken for years. Aromatase inhibitors can be another approach to hormonal-modulating treatment. These change the impact of estrogen in the body, often blocking it. They too can have menopausal-like side effects and are often used in the short term. Dopamine agonists can slow down the ability of endometriotic tissue to form new blood vessels and survive. More experimental options, such as selective estrogen receptor modulators (SERMs) and selective progesterone receptor modulators (SPRMs), are less commonly used.

When I speak about these options, people tend to have two common reactions: 1) *Why is it always more hormones?* and 2) *Why does it*

* In 2021, a group of scientists published a thorough systematic review of the scientific literature, scouring decades of research, and found only nine human and twelve animal published studies specifically testing diet as an intervention to *treat* endometriosis. Only two of the studies are randomized trials that directly compare diet to hormones or other treatments. When supplement companies claim "clinical testing" or "clinically proven," that does not mean actual scientific research.

seem complicated, with side effects and all of that? As I hope I've made clear, the gynecologic organs *are* hormonal organs. When we have conditions that go wrong, it makes sense that our treatments are also hormonal. That is the most direct pathway to correcting what has gone off-kilter. I think we have such a strong aversion to hormones because they are so gender-coded. In common use, *hormones* almost always means something related to women, and if women's health interventions aren't completely "natural," they're somehow intrinsically evil and sinister. If women can't find relief using a natural remedy, they should just suffer because the malfunction is probably their fault anyway. Let's break free of this. It's misogyny, pure and simple. As to the second question of why it seems complicated? Because it is. Like every other organ in the body, the gynecologic organs are complicated. Like every other biological tissue we have, the endometrium is complex. In fact, it's quite a gift how hormonally sensitive the endometrium is—because we can use something already innate to our bodies, estrogen, and modulate its level to treat a disease and achieve major improvement in pain and quality of life. That's about as natural as it gets.

The race to find new treatments for endometriosis is on. Researchers are looking to see how to target endometrial cells' ability to migrate and turn that off, how to make the cell lesions die spontaneously (apoptosis) so they go away without surgery, how to prevent their inflammatory chain of events that causes so much damage, and how to pause the abnormal gene expression that starts the entire process to begin with.

SURGICAL REMOVAL OF ENDOMETRIOSIS

Before Mya was given a prescription for Lupron, she had surgery. For the migrated endometrial tissue that has simply grown too big to respond adequately to estrogen changes, we have the option to remove it. Surgery removes the primary cause of the cascading inflammation and pain cycle, the instigator and agitator. There may still be inflammation and scarring left behind, but without repeatedly adding gas to the fire, these also might die out. As it was in Mya's case, when a patient has a diagnostic laparoscopy, they often give their surgeon consent to move forward with "destruction of endometriosis lesions" as treatment if that's deemed appropriate.

Not all endometriosis is created equal. Some women may have just a few small lesions on their uterine surface, while others have lesions so extensive that their pelvic organs are essentially frozen in place.* Surprisingly, the extent of lesions does not necessarily correlate to the amount of pain. I have personally excised extensive endometriosis in patients whose only symptom was mild constipation. Others we have taken to the operating room sure we will find that type of frozen pelvis, only to see a few small lesions here and there. The mismatch in symptoms and lesions is frustrating to the patients who want answers and it's frustrating to us as surgeons seeking to heal.

Surgery can put nearby organs at risk. For example, an ovarian endometrioma can be removed and every care will be taken to preserve the ovary, but this is not always possible. If endometrial lesions have entrapped the ureter—the tube that drains the kidneys—and caused a partial blockage, this can ultimately compromise kidney function. A skilled surgeon can remove these lesions and improve kidney function, but success is not guaranteed. Bowel lesions can be carefully stripped, but severe cases can require partial bowel excisions. Same with the bladder and everywhere else endometriosis shows up. These are important, often technically difficult surgeries, and they are deeply undervalued by the biomedical healthcare system. Surgeons who perform these operations use small incisions to facilitate faster recovery and avoid increasing inflammation, a technique that can take hours longer in the operating room. These surgeons thoughtfully administer anti-inflammatory and hormonal treatments to prolong the surgical benefit. These surgeries are often done by MIGS gynecologists or gynecologic oncologists because we've had significantly more training on complex pelvic surgery. De-

---

* Surgeons call this a *frozen pelvis* because of the buildup of scar tissue that prevents the surrounding organs from being able to move.

spite our highly specialized efforts, these procedures are poorly reimbursed, reflecting the systemic devaluation of women's healthcare.* This disinvestment in women's health has profound impacts on all of our lives.

Women who have undergone multiple surgeries, failed medical treatments, and who don't want to bear biological children can choose to remove their ovaries. Ovarian removal (oophorectomy) is a nearly curative treatment because endometriosis is fueled by estrogen, and the main source of estrogen is the ovaries. However, individual outcomes can vary, with recent evidence showing ovarian removal is beneficial for some, but not all. Taking out the womb, in addition to the ovaries, uproots the source of the endometrial-like tissue, and when adenomyosis is present (up to 30 percent of the time), it also removes a source of significant pain. My colleagues who specialize in endometriosis (I do not) caution against implying that ovarian and uterine removal is foolproof treatment for endometriosis. They have seen it come back after these surgeries, and endometriotic tissue can stimulate its own growth. And, as a gynecologic oncologist who has seen endometriosis destroy entire sections of bowel, bladder, and more, *I* think it is reasonable to consider ovarian and uterine removal in severe cases *before* these other organs are compromised. *I* am biased by instances where endometriosis has totally decimated a woman's insides. And *they* are biased by the cases they have where women still had pain after surgery. Choosing surgery is a highly personal decision and getting more than one opinion can help you decide for yourself. Choosing surgery is not a failure. Every person is capable of weighing the potential risks, their own family history, and choosing a future that is best for them.

Nearly one in five hysterectomies in the United States are to treat endometriosis. In the research I've completed with my colleague,

* In fact, procedures specific to female reproductive anatomy are *systematically* reimbursed lower than male-specific procedures. Getting into the financial data on this will enrage you. A doctor gets 45 percent more money to biopsy a penis than to biopsy a vagina. They get nearly 150 percent more to remove a lesion on the penis than to remove a lesion in the vagina. Dr. Jocelyn Fitzgerald, urogynecologist, is a leading voice and researcher in this area.

friend, and epidemiologist Dr. Whitney Robinson (chapter 4), 11 percent of Black women who had a hysterectomy across ten hospitals in the South had endometriosis documented as the primary indication. This makes me sad. I do not mean to cast what we call *definitive surgery* as negative or as a failure in any way. For many women, choosing a hysterectomy is an empowering act that begins a major shift in their quality of life. In fact, I have rarely come across a woman who was well counseled, well informed, and well prepared that ended up regretting the surgery. (In the absence of even one of these three, there is great potential for dissatisfaction.) But the broader perspective makes me sad because simply, as I've said before, I love the womb. I want as many of us as possible to be able to live our lives with our gynecologic organs intact. And Black women either are not offered or do not utilize *uterine-sparing* options as often as other groups. In our studies, we found Black women have double the severity of symptoms of White women, while receiving no increase in uterine-sparing treatments before hysterectomy. The rate of hysterectomy (for all reasons, not just endometriosis) among Black women is up to 80 percent higher compared to White women in certain age groups. Black women are much, much more likely to have a hysterectomy for treatment. I think it's too often the case that by the time we are finally believed, are finally fed up with the pain and discomfort, there is only one option: Take it all out. I want more freedom for us than that.

After Mya's surgery and her six months of medical therapy, Dr. Taverna-Miller was pleased with the results, and so was Mya. By now, Mya had graduated from college (with honors in public health) and was headed to North Carolina to enter one of the top PhD programs in the country in pursuit of becoming a preeminent cancer epidemiologist. She had also recently been asked to join the board of trustees at Brown University. Her intelligence, tenacity, and leadership skills were being recognized at the highest levels. "I was feeling much better, but I was moving pretty far away. Dr. Taverna-Miller felt I needed a local doctor to follow up with, and I agreed with her." Shortly after moving to campus, Mya set out to find a gynecologist. It was 2016, and she knew her institution had a top-tier medical school and thought nothing of requesting the first gynecologist available for a new patient. These doctors were on faculty at one of the best hospitals in the state. "I was so naive. I didn't even consider it could go badly."

In making her appointment, Mya was meticulous with her medical history and emphasized that she wanted to establish care for endometriosis. During her intake process, she shared that she had recently had surgical treatment and been on a heavy-duty medication for six months and was in recovery. She was doing well but wanted to get acquainted with a new gynecologist who could continue to help her manage her chronic condition. Mya's new doctor greeted her, seemingly without having read any of her history. "She called me a 'healthy twenty-two-year-old with no medical problems.' I was so taken aback." Mya politely tried to remind (or inform) her new doctor of her recent diagnosis, surgery, and treatment and was met with little adjustment to her initial attitude. "The whole visit was so off. By the time we got to the pelvic exam, I was thinking I just needed to get my Pap and get out of there." Mya was on her back, legs in stirrups, attempting to get through this visit to get the healthcare she needed when the doctor decided to bring up a strange topic: Henrietta Lacks.* While she was inserting a speculum into Mya's vagina, using the cytology brush to collect a sample for cervical cancer screening, she decided to gush to Mya about one of the Black women most exploited by the biomedical research industrial complex in history. "I just really appreciate Henrietta Lacks. She really contributed so much to what we know. What a sacrifice." Mya recounts the doctor's words to me as I shake my head. For the first time since we began speaking, she leans forward and puts her hands on her

* This is the Black Baltimore woman who went for healthcare at Johns Hopkins in 1951 and ended up having her cervical tissue biopsied and used for research without her consent. Her cells were special—they were "immortal" and perfect for research, nicknamed *HeLa* cells, and went on to be crucial to decades of scientific discovery. Read more on her and other Black women whose bodies have been vital to scientific discovery in chapter 2, "Origins."

knees to emphasize her next point. "Kemi, I was done. I did not go back to a gynecologist for nearly four years."

I understand why this reference at this precise moment set Mya off. In some ways, the doctor was furthering a legacy of disrespect Black women have faced in seeking medical care. She was also echoing a general disregard of Black women's humanity that has been prevalent throughout history. Angela Davis writes in *Women, Race & Class* about how Black enslaved women in the fields worked under the same expectations of physical labor and productivity as the men. We as Black women never benefited from a gendered assumption of delicateness or fragility. There is a direct through line from antebellum assumptions about the Black woman's body to an early 2000s research study where Black and White actors were asked to present as if they were having a heart attack on camera. Doctors watched the videos and, based on their evaluation, decided if the actors should be sent for urgent cardiac catheterization, a lifesaving procedure. The only group statistically *unlikely* to get referred? Black women. The Black women actors said the same lines as everyone else, but overwhelmingly, they received a different response. Their pain was not seen, so it did not exist.

Mya is a smart, capable, and wildly resilient human being. She had single-handedly taken control of her gynecologic health, become an expert on her own condition, and found quality care despite multiple barriers. She received explicit advice from both loved ones and professionals that she didn't need the care she knew that she did. She was studying to get a PhD in cancer epidemiology, exquisitely aware of the importance of cancer screening, including for cervical cancer, which is why she knew she needed that Pap smear. She knew with her endometriosis that she had a condition that was not curable and needed close care and surveillance. But Mya was also a human being. And she couldn't take it anymore. "I needed a break. I felt better after [Dr. Taverna-Miller's treatment plan], and I was just done." She dutifully requested her birth control refills on time for her contraceptive needs and kept going. Mya had a few pain-free years before her symptoms slowly started to interfere with her life again.

PAIN TREATMENT AND SUPPLEMENTS

The hormonal therapies and surgical interventions I have covered are meant to stop the endometriosis process and therefore improve pain and quality of life. But pain also can and should be addressed directly. Non-medicinal interventions including cognitive behavioral therapy, yoga, and acupuncture have been demonstrated to improve endometriosis pain levels, especially cyclic period pain. For non-cycle-related pelvic pain, *one* scientific study demonstrated a group of nutritional supplements—(vitamins (B6, A, C, E), mineral salts (Ca, Mg, Se, Zn, Fe), lactic ferments, and fish oil (omega-3/6)—were equally as effective as combined hormonal therapy in decreasing non-menstrual pelvic pain after endometriosis surgery. (They were not as effective in decreasing period-associated pain or pain with sex.) There is decent evidence from randomized controlled trials that vitamin C (1000 mg/day) and vitamin E (800–1200 mg/day) supplements, through an antioxidant effect, can improve both chronic pain and the pain related to menstrual cycles in people with endometriosis. (Vitamin D, not so much.) This can be an option for those who can't tolerate NSAIDs or who want to add on to the effect of NSAIDs and other medications. Melatonin is another potential option. Though evidence is more limited, there is one randomized trial where individuals with endometriosis took either melatonin (10 mg) or placebo for eight weeks and rated their pain. Those who took melatonin reported decreased daily pain and reduction in the need for traditional pain medication. As addressed in my exploration of heavy periods (chapter 4, "Heavy Menstrual Bleeding"), we should not overlook the significant impact of over-the-counter anti-inflammatory medications either. For many women, taking these medications means the difference between being couch-ridden and being able to leave the house. And many women need more. About 30 percent of women diagnosed with endometriosis will eventually develop pelvic pain that is untreatable with standard methods. Complex pain management involves many different players, including specialists who can address both inflammatory and neuropathic (nerve-based) pain, pelvic floor physical therapists, and mental health support. Specialists who can help address lifestyle factors, including diet, exercise, sleep, and stress levels, are incredibly helpful as well.*

When Mya's pain came back, she wasn't surprised. She knew this was a possibility, and she reluctantly went back to the medical system, looking for care. This time, she found a gynecologist through campus health services. Thankfully, she again found an empathetic ear, someone who believed her. "She wasn't an endometriosis specialist, but she had experience treating it, and we really worked together to minimize my symptoms." Mya brightens as she tells me this, and I incorrectly assume we are through the worst of her stories. Mya shifted through different formulations of combination estrogen-progesterone medications and ultimately switched to what is called *continuous use* for menstrual suppression. She would take them straight through the month, not breaking to have a monthly bleed. All these changes helped her, until they didn't.

"It was better, but it was also getting worse over the long term. I wasn't bleeding anymore, so that helped, but I was still getting pain, like clockwork when my cycle was due, for five to seven days. And I was starting to have the same problems: staying in the house, missing out on social gatherings, pain with sex." Both she and her doctor were starting to suspect she might need surgery again. It was now early 2021, COVID had taken its toll on our healthcare systems, and all medical visits were still being done via virtual audio-video platforms unless meeting in person was absolutely necessary. Mya had secured a virtual appointment with a MIGS gynecologist based in the academic medical center. The way Mya slows her speaking immediately puts me on edge. I ask if she needs a break, and she declines. I brace myself for what is coming. "I remember she logged on late to the Zoom room. I understood, though. Clinicians are busy, and I knew already from doctor friends by then how crazy the scheduling can be, not having enough time for each person and all that. So, she

* The brevity here is not a dismissal. It's simply a large-enough topic to be a whole separate book, and this one is focused on gynecology.

apologized and it was fine. She said she was late because she was going through my records. I had uploaded everything—my surgery notes, my pathology report, the pictures, everything ahead of time. She had gone through my records and she opened the visit by telling me she didn't believe I had endometriosis." Mya pauses, and I can't suppress my small gasp. "She said that she didn't believe a 'community doctor' knew enough to diagnose it and that it was wrong for her to have given me the Lupron. She didn't care what I had to say. She prescribed me a muscle relaxant and declined to discuss surgery or any other options."

Mya struggled to put into words the emotions she felt in that moment. She had the gold standard for diagnosis, a surgically resected tissue that had been analyzed by pathologists under a microscope and confirmed to be endometriosis, proving that she had the condition. She had the classic symptoms and had even improved after receiving treatments associated with the diagnosis. She was reaching out for help as an informed person with both lived experience and knowledge about her disease, and she was dismissed. Again. She was angry and disappointed in the elitism, she told me. She felt her diagnosis was being summarily dismissed simply because her surgeon, Dr. Taverna-Miller, had been based in the community and not an academic institution. In academic medical centers, there is a pervasive view that community-based physicians cannot deliver the same quality of care as these centers of higher learning.

Academic medical centers are expected to be at the forefront of new knowledge, technologies, and research in all areas of medicine. It is true that it can take time for updates in care practices to reach community-based doctors who are busy clinically, but not necessarily attending lectures on the newest discoveries. On the other hand, the idea that community-based physicians and hospitals, that by far provide the vast majority of all medical care in the United States, are inherently less competent is wrong and reeks of the elitism that plagues academic settings.

Mya's diagnosis was dismissed because it didn't come from an academic surgeon. Mya felt a strong sense of defense for Dr. Taverna-Miller, the community-based gynecologist who believed her. "It sounds kind of wild to say, [but] I don't go hard for very many White women in my life," Mya says with a laugh. "I will go hard for my initial surgeon." After the appointment at which her beloved doctor's diagnosis and treatment plan were undermined, Mya turned off the Zoom, dismissed and dejected. "I continued to quite honestly suffer for the rest of grad school . . . staying inside . . . not doing anything. My pain was off the charts." Despite her monthly bleeding being suppressed, Mya was still experiencing severe pain with her cycles. Each month, the endometriotic tissue that had built up again in her pelvis was still bleeding, inflamed, and painful. She spent about a week each month confined to her apartment, and a few days after that recovering slowly until she could emerge again. She graduated with her PhD in cancer epidemiology, with honors, on time.

As a highly sought-after candidate, Mya skipped the postdoc training fellowships recent PhD graduates often take to further their training. Instead, she secured a coveted tenure-track faculty position directly after graduation, this time at Vanderbilt University in Nashville, Tennessee. She had gotten engaged while in graduate school and was excited about this new phase in her life. Having given up entirely on any improvement in her healthcare while in school, she waited until she moved to Nashville and settled in before looking for a new doctor. She would not go for the first available appointment again. And she had sworn off academic medical centers, still angry at the dismissal of her diagnosis. "I specifically looked for a Black primary care doctor who would take my insurance. I just couldn't go straight back to gynecologists." She found someone and dutifully filled out the litany of new-patient questionnaires to start her first visit. Mya's new doctor reviewed her answers and opened this visit quite differently. "I can see that you probably don't feel as well as you would like," she said. "Let's talk about that."* It was such a simple and powerful statement, from one Black woman who could truly see another. They went through Mya's symptoms, and the doctor narrowed in on one that Mya herself had not clocked as unusual: her

* To my physician colleagues—I love this. Isn't it a powerful and open way to hear the truth of someone's experience?

urinary frequency. "She was like, so, I want to talk about how you have to pee four times in an hour," Mya said, laughing. "I had not even noticed that was odd. I just figured that's what happens when you drink water." Her doctor did notice that this was unusual, especially at Mya's young age of twenty-six. She recommended a referral to someone she knew and trusted, a urogynecologist who specialized in pelvic floor disorders, including incontinence and prolapse. Trusting her new primary care doctor, Mya went.

Her urogynecologist was respectful and curious. They spoke in detail about Mya's challenges with painful sex, locating the when, where, and how of her symptoms both during their discussions and with a slow and thorough pelvic exam. "She got fully in the nitty-gritty, detailed questions, which were so helpful for me because I was thinking of my body in a way I hadn't previously, even though I had been living with endometriosis for quite some time." With Mya's continued worsening pain symptoms and her new urinary symptoms, the specialist recommended a second surgery for endometriosis. It was scheduled, as was a routine preoperative ultrasound to help map out her anatomy. After the scan, Mya received a surprising phone call. "It was one of the most terrifying phone calls I have ever had." They found something surprising on her scan, a mass near her fallopian tube. The doctor knew it had to be one of three things: an ectopic pregnancy, a fibroid, or cancer. The office asked her to get a pregnancy test right away. Mya is sober during this recollection. "I felt so alone. I was in this new city by myself, I didn't really know anyone yet. My husband had just gotten deployed. And my mom had just passed a few months prior." Mya's mother had been diagnosed with a liver condition during Mya's last years in graduate school. Her decline was rapid, and she died soon after Mya moved to Nashville. Mya remembers driving to the CVS to pick up the pregnancy test and feeling a "deep sense of loneliness that I wouldn't wish on my worst enemy." Her test was negative. She was left with two possibilities: a fibroid or cancer.

Mya found a co-worker to drive her to surgery and checked in to the preoperative area alone. She had already activated a special process to contact a deployed service member in case of a family emergency. If anything went wrong, her husband would be notified. Her surgeon was running behind by several hours. The initial nursing and anesthesia teams she met had left. Their shifts ended while Mya was still waiting. "I was sobbing my eyes out in part because when I was in that boat several years prior . . . my mom was there. And there I was sitting, basically in the same position, six years later, and I had nobody." Eventually, Mya's surgeon would appear, apologetic about having run behind because of an operation involving a surprising case of "complex fibroids." Mya would have preferred not to know that tidbit, as it set her even more on edge.

She woke from the surgery without complications. The findings? Mya's endometriosis was indeed back. This time, it had also coated her bladder, explaining her new urinary symptoms. The mass on her fallopian tube was the best-case scenario—an oddly placed fibroid. It was removed. Prior to her waking up, as they had discussed, her surgeon placed a progesterone IUD in her uterus, for continued medical treatment after the surgery. Mya was relieved. And most importantly, pain-free again.

I asked Mya how she felt about the surgical findings. "I got bowel issues. I got bladder issues. I got uterus—" Her laughter interrupts her words. "I can't even pick a struggle." Mya is graceful and humorous, her head unbowed. At the time of our interview, in 2024, Mya is still pain-free. She's moved back to North Carolina and is in her second year at a new faculty position. She hasn't reestablished gynecologic care. "Quite honestly, I don't know when I'll go back to the gynecologist. I'm overdue for my Pap, but I feel fine now. I have my IUD, [so] I'm good for a couple more years."

I ask Mya what she imagines her life might have been like without endometriosis. "I would have so much less experience with the healthcare system, probably in a good way. I would have had far fewer negative health encounters. I am a highly educated, high-income Black woman. And I don't trust the healthcare system, because of all I have been through."

I remind Mya of the specific accomplishments that have led to her self-identification as "highly educated and high income." She was the first in her family to go to college. She graduated from an Ivy League college with honors and joined the Brown University Board of Trustees. She earned her master's and then PhD degree in cancer epidemiology after matriculating into a top-five PhD program. Mya married a wonderful person and deeply felt love, and she co-managed her mother's terminal illness. She secured a prestigious faculty position and immediately won competitive research grants. She is an associate editor of a major medical journal, influential in her field. As expected, she is buoyed by hearing her accolades reflected at her. "You know, laying it all out like that . . . it's amazing that I made it this far and I still have so much joy." I'm curious what brings her joy right now. "Spending time outside, hearing the birds sing, feeling the sun on my face, and practicing aerial arts."

Like the endometriotic tissue that has caused her so much trouble over the course of her life, Mya is powerful and tenacious. As a scientist and collector of stories, I am somehow inspired and enthralled by both the woman and the condition she is surviving. In the endometrial cells' ability to migrate and transform themselves, I see echoes of Mya's experience and the experiences of Black women more broadly. We journey from where we are told we belong, the small boxes we are told to fit into. Instead, we take the back door out, we inspire others to want to be like us, and some of us make big leaps into worlds unknown, knowing we will co-create our success with whatever the new reality brings. Like the cells that sometimes plague us internally, Black women learn to adapt. These adaptations ensure our temporary survival but are painful, destructive, and often hidden unless we scream in pain about it and hope somebody who can help believes us.

Whether there is debilitating pain or not, whether your pelvis is frozen or not, endometriosis matters. The more we understand the condition, the more vigilant we can be about assessing our bodies' signals—and the more knowledgeable we can be about how to navigate diagnostic and treatment options with confidence.

When endometriosis is diagnosed early, patients have the most treatment options with the fewest long-term, permanent consequences. Unfortunately, research tells us that when endometriosis starts in adolescence, we are more likely to delay seeking evaluation and more likely to normalize abnormal levels of pain. A teenager with endometriosis will wait an average of three and a half years from the time symptoms start to getting her first consultation. After that, it will be an average of another three years before she gets a diagnosis. Under these circumstances, she is likely to have six and a half years of untreated and unnecessary inflammation, internal bleeding, and pain. Our girls and young women deserve better. If any of the following apply, and especially if two or more are a yes, it is worth speaking to a gynecologist about the possibility of endometriosis and potential treatments.

- Painful menarche—a first period that is painful and requires pain medications
- Painful periods that routinely require bed rest, causing you to miss school or work
- Nausea or vomiting that accompanies painful cycles
- Pelvic pain that happens outside of your period and lasts for days
- Painful sex
- Close relationship between bowel movements and menstrual pain. Often pain gets noticeably worse or significantly better after bowel movements.
- Painful and frequent urination during menstrual cycles

Endometriosis will rarely kill you, but it will create debilitating pain and suffering that you can feel and no one else can see. Your relief depends on you deciding you deserve better, finding a doctor who believes your pain, and choosing, despite all valid concerns about the medical system, to seek treatment. In part 3 of this book, we will cover, in detail, what good gynecologic care actually looks like.

CHAPTER 6

FIBROIDS

The Neglected Womb

On the first day of my general surgery rotation in medical school, the operating room I stepped into had one case—a Whipple. I don't remember if I was assigned or if we got to choose, but I had no idea what I was walking into. A Whipple is among the most complex of abdominal operations. The goal is to remove tumors from the head of the pancreas. There are many critical structures and organs in the way, and you have to take them apart and put them back together to get the job done. The surgery lasted over fifteen hours. We took one break. The surgeons told me many times I could leave and go home. But there was no way I was leaving that operating room, no matter how hungry I felt or how much my arms shook from the fatigue of holding retracting instruments for hours. My commitment to this patient continued long after the surgery ended. I followed him from his time in the ICU, through to the regular inpatient ward, and then to his discharge. This sometimes meant taking pre–5:00 A.M. trains to work, even though I was genuinely apprehensive about being alone as a young woman on the subway platform in what felt like the middle of the night. I swallowed the fear. The entire time I cared for this White man, he hurled disparaging insults at me that made my skin crawl. I ignored it. I was simply following a tired and dangerous script of Black womanhood. But it worked. I earned honors during that rotation. The adjectives my supervisors used to describe me were "excellent" and "indefatigable." Pushing the limit of my physical, mental, and emotional well-being was a core skill in my achievement bag. Self-neglect was my badge of courage.

Ten years later, during the testing I had for my infertility workup, a transvaginal ultrasound had revealed I had a fibroid in the muscle wall of the uterus. It was small, under 4 cm, and to me, asymptomatic. From my training, I knew it wasn't stopping me from getting pregnant, so it didn't really matter to me. I knew the narrative: Fibroids were benign tumor growths that were harmless unless they created symptoms, in which case, you could remove them. Unknowingly following the script of disassociation and neglect, I put it out of my mind. I did achieve pregnancy via IVF, and I certainly didn't think about it then. My focus was on going to work, continuing my training, and falling asleep on the couch within a few minutes of getting home each night. It was an early morning in my second trimester when I woke up with pain. It was a dull, subtle throbbing. But I didn't have any bleeding, which would suggest a miscarriage, so I ignored it. I went to work, saw patients in clinic, wrote up clinical notes, and kept going. I drank a bit more water.

The following week, I was assigned to the operating room. I was still hurting. I remember being annoyed that I couldn't just take ibuprofen, my usual medication to dull pain, because I knew it could compromise fetal kidney development. After two days, I was doubled over in pain when walking into the house each night, hissing whenever

I would accidentally bump into a piece of furniture or even bend over too far, as my pelvic area had become quite tender. My spouse was done with my reassurances when he realized I was avoiding standing up straight because it hurt too much. He demanded I call to get an urgent doctor's visit. "But I'm not bleeding," I said. I ticked through other symptoms. "I don't have a fever. I'm not nauseated." An urgent visit would pull me out of surgery and inconvenience my colleagues. I wanted to be a good team player. The fact that I was "just" hurting didn't seem worth the disruption. My spouse is a preternaturally Zen person. This is for sure why we work together. He harbors a laissez-faire attitude and rarely gets angry, born of his deep respect of other people's autonomy. He doesn't tell anyone what to do. So, when he insisted and would not let the topic drop, I agreed to see the doctor.

I called for an appointment that day and showed up in my surgical scrubs, fully planning to go back to work afterward. After hearing my story, the physician, a maternal fetal medicine specialist, did a bedside scan, using an ultrasound probe to take a look at my uterus. As I rolled up my scrub top and rolled down my pants to bare my belly, I gritted my teeth. I didn't like being vulnerable like that, especially at work. When I put my scrubs on, the rest of my body disappeared from my consciousness. I used my brain to think, my arms to operate, and my legs to get me around. The rest was gone. This was a strange unveiling. I was once again a Black woman with a pelvic problem. Though I knew much more of what to expect than when I was seventeen at that first appointment when the cold jolt of the speculum was my introduction to gynecology, the discomfort this time was just as palpable. Was it the sense of being watched and judged that stoked my unease? The part of me that learned as a child that my pain was likely to be viewed with suspicion and dismissal was livid to be put back in such a vulnerable position. My thoughts ran on a loop: I wasn't bleeding. I was probably overreacting. The pain wasn't that bad. I could still work.

I stayed still, submitting to the scan. After confirming the fetal heartbeat looked fine, he scanned around to see more of my uterus. After a few seconds, I nearly jumped off the table in pain. He found the source: my fibroid.

While once it had seemed unobtrusive and insignificant on a scan, it was now inflamed with the telltale signs of necrosis, meaning the cells were dying from the inside out. Fibroid cells sometimes cannot adjust to the quick and profound hormonal shifts during pregnancy. They die off and release prostaglandins that create a whole bunch of inflammation. It is very painful and can prompt uterine contractions and even pregnancy loss. Despite being an ob-gyn, despite knowing I had a fibroid, despite learning about the symptoms caused by degenerating fibroids in the course of my training, my disassociation and neglect of my own fibroid was so strong that I had never considered this diagnosis. So, when I hear women speak about simply not thinking about their fibroids, I understand fully.

At the appointment, the doctor reminded me that stopping the inflammatory process was key to both pain relief and preventing further escalation that could threaten my pregnancy. So, despite the risks, I was started on a high dose of NSAIDs and an aggressive hydration regimen. He also strongly suggested I go home and rest. I stumbled, slowly, out of that visit. I had finally stopped trying to push through the pain, which had increased as a result of the exam. I allowed my spouse to support me as we walked back to the car, leaning on his offered arm. I followed doctors' orders and didn't do much for the next forty-eight hours other than sleep, hydrate, and take NSAIDs. I prayed my baby's kidneys would be okay and that this wouldn't cause problems like low amniotic fluid in the future.

On a Friday, I went back to work so I could participate in our weekly Tumor Board, a conference where we re-

viewed cases of the week and discussed treatment plans. I could move around more easily but was still slow with walking. As my colleagues zoomed ahead of me going from one building to another, I felt embarrassed. I did not have a mode in which I could be weak or vulnerable at work. I felt unmoored without my default tactic of neglecting my body in favor of hard work. And although treatment had helped me in that I felt better and was more functional, it also left me feeling helpless. This thing was still inside me and could still create problems for me, and the only definitive solution was to cut it out. I put it out of my mind. I still do.

The earliest written reports of fibroids refer to them as "uterine stones." In the 1860s, the term *leiomyoma* was introduced, but the original second-century A.D. phrase is especially descriptive. Fibroids are noncancerous tumors within the uterus. They are sometimes inconvenient, causing someone who lives with fibroids to bleed excessively, appear bulky around their midsection, or perhaps experience pain with sex. But they're not lethal for the vast majority of patients. They are something to endure, clinicians have long advised, and Black women have far more practice than others when it comes to learning to live with these stones in our wombs.

Fibroids are common. They are found in women and people with a uterus from all backgrounds, but they do not impact us equally. This is a condition for which the racial disparities are clear and the differences start early. Among young women, with an average age of twenty-five and no prior fibroid diagnosis, an ultrasound found fibroids in 26 percent of Black women. The number was only 7 percent for White women. By age fifty, a full 50 percent of all Black women will have a significant and symptomatic fibroid. Half of us. Even these staggering percentages are perhaps too low, reflecting only those women who report their symptoms to a provider or in a research study. This erases those who are asymptomatic but may have problems down the line. When we consider *all* fibroids—symptomatic or not—the vast majority, 80 percent, of Black women will have at least one.

To understand what fibroids are and how they grow, we have to remember how the womb is structured (see chapter 3, "The Basics"). The thickest part of the uterus is made up of the middle layer, the myometrium. In Latin, *myo* means "muscle." The myometrium is made up of sheets of muscle cells, or *myocytes,* woven together with structural tissue called *extracellular matrix,* or ECM for short. This layer of the womb powers the contraction and relaxation of the uterus, movements that occur in response to hormonal and neural signals.

This middle layer of the womb also contains *stem cells,* which hold the genetic history and the instructions required to make new muscle cells. These round blue cells look different from the surrounding pink muscle tissue. We need new muscle cells as we age, if the uterus is damaged and needs to repair itself, and during pregnancy. The stem cells activate in these times of need. As evidence of the layer's beautiful interdependence, it is the mature muscle cells that signal back to the stem cells when it's time to replicate—that is, to make more of the stem cells themselves.

Fibroids occur when the myometrium loses that intricate system of coordination and purpose. Something goes wrong with the muscle stem cell replication. A mistake in the process creates a new myometrial stem cell that *looks* normal but isn't. It starts making new uterine muscle cells, and those aren't normal either. These new myocytes are disordered in three key ways. First, they grow in random islands instead of in the ordered sheets needed for muscles to contract properly. They form clumps that don't line up with the normal uterine muscle cells, and this awkward ball of muscle strains the smooth muscles around it. That can be painful in a contracting or growing uterus, such as during a menstrual cycle or pregnancy. Second, the new muscle cells developing from the damaged stem cell also make *much* more of that structural ECM tissue than is needed, making this disordered ball of muscle larger and harder. Third, these new muscle cells start making their *own* estrogen, which prompts growth. Fibroid cells have *aromatase,* an enzyme protein that can make estrogen. Estrogen alone doesn't change fibroids. Estrogen makes the fibroids more sensitive to progesterone, which sends the fibroid into overdrive, staying alive and growing in ways that mess up typical uterine function. Luckily, fibroids very rarely acquire more mutations, which is why they are considered "benign tumors" in medicine. They almost never turn into cancer.

Why do fibroids grow inside of us? There are many factors both within the body and outside of it that influence your risk of developing fibroids. In the Black Women's Health Study (BWHS), nearly sixty thousand Black women were followed for over twenty-five years, reporting information on their lifestyles and medical events every two years. Given how much misinformation abounds regarding fibroid causes and treatments, I believe it is worth spending some time telling you what the data actually shows for Black women, specifically. Here are some of the results that are clear and consistent: Fibroid risk is higher the earlier you get your first period. Black women, and other women of color, get periods earlier in life and so start off at higher risk. Fibroid risk is lower, overall, for those who have birthed children compared to those who haven't. The number of children does not matter. The number of miscarriages or abortions you have had has no relationship to your future risk of fibroids. Whether you breastfeed (or chestfeed) or not, for whatever length of time, has no relationship to fibroid risk. (Do not fall for the guilt trips!)

Let's get into some more controversial topics like birth control and obesity. First, there is no consistent connection between birth control pills and developing fibroids. No, there isn't. You can find studies, not focused on Black women, that show that hormonal birth control increases fibroids and those that show that it decreases fibroids and many that are in between. In the Black Women's Health Study, they were comprehensive—they looked at type of birth control, duration of use, strength of the hormonal dosing, type of hormones included, and more. They got all up in these women's business, and there was only one factor that was *weakly* associated with increased fibroid risk—taking an oral birth control pill before age seventeen.* That is it. Here is what I think is happening with this birth control and fibroid discourse. Most folks start hormonal birth control sometime in their twenties, and we know from Dr. Erica Marsh's data and others', this is the same decade we start seeing an increase in fibroid development and growth in the womb. This does not mean one causes the other. And in fact, when we study thousands of Black women who have never taken any hormonal birth control, *they are also developing and growing fibroids during this time.* That is what the data, covering Black women across the country for decades, shows. There are so many interventions needed to help Black women with the incredible burden of fibroids in their lives, and repeating myths that blame birth control is not one of them.

What about body size? The Black Women's Health Study also researched this in many ways: BMI at eighteen years old, current BMI, waist-to-hip ratio, weight change over time, waist and hip circumference, and height. This was a very thorough way to look at this question—and remember this data is *all* from Black women. Here is what they found: The only parameter that consistently increased risk of fibroid development was weight gain since age eighteen, *among folks who had given birth* (*parous* in medical terms). For those who had not given birth (*nulliparous*), there was almost no influence of any body size parameter on fibroid development.†

How about data that is actionable right now? Increased physical activity decreases fibroid risk. Black women with seven hours per week or more of vigorous physical activity (at any body size) have *40 percent decreased fibroid risk* compared to those with less than two hours per week. And it's not all or none. Four hours is better than two hours, for example. Why? The theory is that exercise is known to decrease circulating sex hormone levels and increase the proteins that bind up estrogen—further lowering estrogen levels, specifically in the luteal phase of premenopausal women. As the popular phrase goes, movement is medicine.

* Weakly, meaning 10–20 percent increased risk overall. For example, if normal risk is 10 percent, then a 20 percent increase from normal is 12 percent.

† So, if you see anyone—doctor, holistic healer, or otherwise—making sweeping claims about obesity and fibroids, be wary.

What about diet? Increased intake of fruits and vegetables, increased dietary calcium, and increased vitamin D levels all correlate to lower fibroid risk. In nonhuman animal experiments, lycopene, found chiefly in tomatoes, was noted to be protective against fibroids, but when follow-up human studies were done, this correlation did not bear out.* And then there is soy. Soy contains isoflavones, which are phyto-estrogens, or plant-derived compounds that are structurally similar to human estrogen. This means these compounds can, theoretically, either mimic—*or block*—the effect of estrogen in our bodies. In premenopausal women, soy acts more like an estrogen blocker. (It competes with estrogen for the same receptor, so your uterine cells get less actual estrogen.) In postmenopausal women (who have much lower estrogen levels), soy can have more estrogen-mimicking effects. What does all of this mean? It means that soy does *not* increase risk of fibroids. We know because from 1997 to 2007, more than twenty-two thousand women in the BWHS participated in the research that measured number of soy servings per week with subsequent uterine fibroid development. The results? No effect. There are some things we take into our bodies, however, that do increase fibroid risk. Having a high dietary glycemic index (lots of simple sugars in your diet), alcohol consumption (especially beer), and dark-meat fish are correlated with increased fibroid risk.†

* Human studies are important. We are not mice, rabbits, hamsters, or chimps. We have to study things in humans.

† I have intentionally left off the data from dairy and meat intake because, frankly, it's confusing, and maybe I'm not being brave enough in countering the popular message about vegan diets controlling fibroids. Here is the data: In the BWHS, dairy intake *decreased* risk of fibroids. Yes, decreased. I think this is due to the calcium intake. In a study where they asked women's mothers if they were given soy-based formula as an infant, they found a slight *increase* in fibroids in those who had received soy formula at less than two months of age for at least six months. I think this is because infants usually get soy formula because of other digestive issues—and that inflammatory state may be more of the culprit. We don't have it figured out yet. In terms of other animal products—there is no association between red meat or poultry meat and fibroid risk. The one animal-based fat that is associated with increased risk is fish—specifically the omega-3 fatty acid docosahexaenoic acid. This counters what we know scientifically about omega-3s being excellent for working against tumor growth. Right now, one theory is that this finding represents environmental pollution—that the fish being consumed contain pollutants that increase the fibroid risk, not the omega-3s themselves. It's not worked out yet. I may stop eating fish, though.

SUMMARY OF DATA FROM THE BLACK WOMEN'S HEALTH STUDY ON FIBROIDS

Associated with INCREASED Fibroid Risk	Associated with DECREASED Fibroid Risk
High dietary glycemic index and glycemic load (especially those < 35 years old)	More than 2 hours/week of vigorous daily exercise (at any body size)
Weight gain (20+ pounds since 18 years old, if given birth)	Intake of fruits and vegetables
Alcohol (specifically > 7 beers/ week)	Intake of vitamin D and calcium
Younger age at first period	Older age at first giving birth
NOT ASSOCIATED with Fibroid Risk	
Body size (among those who haven't given birth)	Number of abortions or miscarriages
Most hormonal birth control	Amount of lactation (breast- or chestfeeding)

The vitamin D data is interesting, and I want us to understand how it works. Vitamin D is a steroid found in two main forms in the body—vitamin D_2 (plants and dairy) and vitamin D_3 (generated in skin from sunlight). Those with darker skin are at increased risk of vitamin D deficiency due to lower levels of absorption from sunlight and the impacts of systemic racism (residential, geographic, and environmental factors) that creates less opportunity to be in sunlight. Similar to the Black Women's Health Study, research in other populations—China, Turkey, Mexico, and Poland, to name a few—have shown a consistent link between lower levels of vitamin D and higher risk of having fibroids. In molecular studies of fibroid cells, vitamin D appears to stop the growth of fibroid cells by 1) reducing their number of estrogen and progesterone receptors and 2) interfering with the creation of new fibrotic tissue. This means vitamin D can be an important component of a holistic approach to fibroid treatment. We will cover how in more detail later in this chapter.

However, like all things disproportionately affecting Black women's health, important non-biological factors related to the impact of racism also influence fibroid development. Severe chronic physiologic stress and moderate daily stress—as measured by validated surveys given to thousands of Black women—both increase fibroid risk. I was amazed by a study that focused on "anger squelching." This refers to a practice all Black women know well—"feeling the need to squelch or swallow strong feelings of anger." I zeroed in on this study because we know Black women are constantly at risk for being labeled the Angry Black Woman. We are the people who must overly police our tone and our diction to avoid being perceived as aggressive and even violent. We are required to learn how to suppress our anger as a basic survival mechanism in this society.

But this anger squelching we do to survive is not without cost, specifically to our wombs. Black women with more episodes of this anger suppression technique were also more likely to have fibroids. Viewed in this light, that statistic I mentioned that 80 percent of Black women will have fibroids by age fifty doesn't seem far-fetched. Childhood physical, sexual, and emotional abuse also increases fibroid risk later in life by 8–36 percent depending on the severity of the abuse.* Black women who used chemical hair relaxers had a 17 percent increased risk of fibroids, thought to be due to endocrine-disrupting chemicals present in the hair relaxers we use more commonly than others. Air pollution increases risk of fibroids, and Black communities are the most exposed racial group to many forms of air pollution, including the toxins specifically associated with fibroid risk.

* Importantly, children who receive strong emotional support in the face of abuse don't face the same increased risk. Isn't it amazing how much we can interrupt the harms that children are exposed to?

Racism impacts where we live and what we are exposed to. With fibroids, there is a direct association between the racism Black women experience and their risk of developing the condition. This isn't always the case with health outcomes we assume to be linked to racism. Often the research doesn't bear out a statistically significant relationship. But when it comes to the Black womb the physical, mental, emotional, and environmental stressors of life make themselves manifest, and the correlation is undeniable. We can see this on a large scale, looking at whole communities, and on a small scale, following the story of one woman's life. My desire to zoom in on the particulars led me to Rose, a dynamic and brilliant STEM educator and Black woman from the Caribbean.

Rose is a tall woman with an easy smile. As we sit in an office on the campus of a California university, she tells me about a research paper she's working on. She has a master's and PhD in education, focused on STEM subjects, and is on faculty in a university working with her colleagues on how to best teach the tenets of increasingly complex science to the next generation. In some ways, education is the family business. She is extremely close to her mother, a teacher and administrator at a local high school in their close-knit community. Rose is from a country in the West Indies, and the lilt in her accent is smooth and inviting.

In fourth grade, Rose was selected to be a peer counselor to help prevent a growing problem on her island: teen pregnancy. Rose was proud to be chosen as her class representative. She attended a sex education class where she learned the material she was tasked with sharing with peers. She was shocked when she learned a girl could get pregnant at thirteen. "It was really scare tactics," she says, reflecting on how that outlier scenario was held up as the norm. The other focus of the program was sexually transmitted diseases. She remembers perusing a big yellow book with medical illustrations of the heart, brain, and other organ systems. She looked over the photos of pregnancy and of "venereal diseases," or STIs. She learned and was coached to teach her classmates that abstinence was the way to avoid either of these fateful outcomes. She was eight, maybe nine years old. This was the same year she started her period.

During that sex education program, Rose never learned what a period was or that she herself would begin to bleed. On the day the blood started, she was in her dark blue school uniform. Her mother was still out for the day at work, so it was her grandmother who was home and on the receiving end when Rose asked innocently, "What's this?" The older woman handed Rose a pad and told her how to put it on. It was not until her mother came home from work that Rose received a bit more information. Her mother gave her a stack of pads and explained when to change them and that this bleeding would happen every month. When I ask Rose if her mother explained anything more to her, particularly the connection to pregnancy or how a period feels, she shakes her head. "We didn't really talk about bodies. You know? Even when my mother was diagnosed with cancer, I didn't realize what she had because she wasn't using any body-part language. It was not until several conversations with her about some doctors' visits she was having that I stopped her because I heard a word—*carcinoma*—and finally realized what we were talking about." That would be over twenty years later, and her mother's cancer in question would be a cancer of the womb, similarly shrouded in silence. For now, as a child, Rose had what she needed: information about the typical schedule of menstruation and tools to absorb the blood and keep her school uniform clean.

Rose attended an all-girls Catholic high school, one of the best in her country. She speaks with pride about the diverse socioeconomic backgrounds of the students, whose parents ranged from diplomats to manual laborers. What united them was academic excellence. "If you went to this school, you were going to be somebody. Miss World or a scientist, anything. But something excellent." Now the school uniforms were all white. Rose had some friends who, like her, had gotten their periods on the early side, during blue uniform days. They mostly found one another through context clues. "In the bathroom, you could just tell because people would have their little purses with them. It was like a little club, you know?" Rose doesn't remember her periods being painful or particularly heavy during this time. She was doubling up pads by the time she was twelve or thirteen, for one or two days at the beginning of her cycle before the bleeding faded away without incident. She was also very regular. "You could set the clock to it," she recalls. Swimming was a mandatory class in high school, and Rose was relieved whenever the class coincided with her cycle and she had a reason to not participate. She continued to share information with her schoolmates who were also menstruating. The early conversations in the bathroom among a few girls became a larger, peer-driven network of information. This is when she learned about the pills. These were magic green pills that helped your period go easier, friends told her. Some of them had very difficult periods marked by nausea and vomiting. "They would be laid out," Rose remembers. "That wasn't me." Still, the green pills helped. They took them around the start of their period, and the pain and bleeding were not so bad.

Rose continued excelling in her school, completing her math and science classes along with the required domestic curriculum: sewing, home economics, and other courses geared toward making her a "full woman," as she remembers the adults at school saying. She graduated in 2000 and set off for Hampton University, an HBCU in Virginia. A good friend chose a college nearby, and when they met back home on the island after their first year, she had "become an Afro-Revolutionary," Rose says with a laugh. Her friend railed against colonialism and the everyday racism they both experienced as Black Caribbeans in the United States. Rose's friend also had an important message. "You remember those green pills?" the friend asked. "You have to get off them!" She showed Rose the official name of the pills (Baralgin) and the suspicious history. This medication had been banned in the United States, the UK, and other colonizing countries. In fact, the only places it seemed to still be distributed at the time were in the Caribbean or on the African continent. "I got off that bad boy immediately," Rose says to me with emphasis. The pills had helped with her menstrual pain and bleeding, but that was not worth whatever potential for harm they had on Black women.*

Rose remembers that her periods were not that bad. She majored in chemistry and made her way through undergraduate studies while managing her cycle. This mostly meant watching the calendar and doubling up those pads. Needing multiple heavy pads at one time to make it through a few days of bleeding means her cycle was likely too heavy, but Rose didn't know this. She graduated and began teaching chemistry (and other subjects) at local Virginia colleges. She knew how to break down complicated concepts so students, especially the predominantly Black and Brown students she taught, could understand and truly enjoy science. Her colleagues noticed her outsize skill. "They worked me over until I was convinced to go to grad school." Rose enrolled in a PhD program in science, technology, engineering, and math (STEM) education.

It was there Rose was diagnosed with fibroids. Her bleeding had gotten heavier. She'd moved from doubling up on pads to quadrupling. For the first couple of days of her cycle, she wore two super maxi–size pads in the front of her underwear and two in the back to control her bleeding. Over time, she began feeling weak, and eventually, campus health providers diagnosed her with anemia and started her on iron supplements. An evaluation with a gynecologist and an ultrasound followed. She remembers a White male doctor who sat down with her to discuss her fibroids and her options. He wrote three options down, in cursive, on a small white piece of paper: *myomectomy, uterine artery embolization,* and a third, which she doesn't quite remember. It may have been *ablation*. The doctor suggested a hysterectomy, only if these failed.

* The primary ingredient in Baralgin is metamizole, described as a painkiller and antispasmodic medication. Interestingly, its precise mechanism of action is unknown, but it is thought to interact through the COX-3 enzyme, which affects both prostaglandins (inflammatory molecules) and the central nervous system (pain relief). One serious side effect is agranulocytosis—which is a life-threatening condition when the body stops making white blood cells. As of 2024, the medication is banned in the UK and available only for veterinary use in the United States and Canada. Interestingly, searching drugs.com shows it is still available throughout the Caribbean.

Then he told her about a clinical trial for which she was eligible. Rose heard alarm bells. "Something about the way he was being so persuasive just sounded off to me. I had been taking ethics in research classes in grad school; I knew something about this." She had learned about the importance of informed consent, avoiding pressure when offering enrollment in clinical trials, and transparency about the design and leadership of a study. She asked him directly if he was the principal investigator, or leader of the study, and if so, why did he not disclose that when speaking with her about it up front? "He immediately backed up, and a nurse finished the visit," she says. Rose was upset and wary. "Like, talk about the issue. Don't bring your study in here. . . . What are you trying to get out of this?" she thought. Though I already know where this story is going to end, I'm moved by now two episodes in Rose's womb-care journey where she experienced fear and distrust of medicine. The green pills that helped her seemed to have a nefarious distribution pattern to Black and Brown countries. The gynecologist she was appropriately referred to botched an attempt to discuss research, pushing and not disclosing his role, clearly not realizing how fearful Rose was about her new diagnosis. These moments matter—in Rose's life and the lives of so many women who begin their womb-care experience negatively. Rose noticed that the doctor had mentioned centimeters regarding her fibroid size, and so she assumed that meant they were small. *Okay,* she thought. *I can use these three options if they get big, but I'm fine for now. I can manage.* The nurse that came afterward had a better bedside manner. She told Rose how she could use ibuprofen to help her symptoms and walked her through the appropriate dosing schedule for heavy menstrual bleeding. Rose started that and immediately experienced some improvement. There was no further follow-up about her fibroids. Rose would have to feel like she was dying before the topic was brought up again.

The symptoms people experience from fibroids depend on the size and position of any given fibroid in their uterus. Around a third of people with fibroids will ultimately have severe symptoms, and this is much more likely to be true for Black women. Why? Black women's fibroids start earlier in life and are greater in number and larger in size than those found in other groups. For Black women, fibroids start growing in the uterus five to ten years earlier than for White women. They grow at the same rate by race, but Black women have a head start, and ours continue to grow for a longer time.

Four out of five women with symptomatic fibroids have altered bleeding patterns as a primary symptom. This bleeding can drain the body of vital blood, leading to iron deficiency, anemia, and the fatigue that accompanies those depleted states.* Fibroids cause issues with bleeding in two ways: 1) If they are located near or inside the inner wall of the uterus, they will disrupt this tissue and prevent the uterine contraction needed to stop bleeding during a cycle; and 2) on a molecular level, they secrete proteins that interfere with the womb's ability to regulate bleeding correctly, thus causing heavy bleeding, irregular bleeding, and/or spotting in between periods.

Fibroids also create "bulk" symptoms, which include pelvic pressure, back or abdominal pain from muscle strain, persistent bloating, or a fullness sensation. This happens when large or sensitively placed fibroids exert pressure in the body. In a large study of 1,384 women with symptomatic fibroids and undergoing some kind of treatment, 74 percent had pelvic pressure, 73 percent had bloating, and 44 percent appeared pregnant because of their fibroids. Fibroids that push against the bladder can increase urinary frequency, and those that push against the bowels can cause constipation. Fibroids can also cause pain. Forty-three percent of women with symptomatic fibroids report painful sex, 43 percent report pelvic pain in general, and 11 percent have non-menstrual pain associated with fibroids.

Finally, fibroids impact fertility. Large fibroids can distort the uterine cavity and result in poor embryo implantation so a potential pregnancy is lost. Five percent of women with fibroids have a history of multiple miscarriages. Fibroids in the lower uterus and cervix can obstruct the birth canal and prevent a healthy vaginal birth. In preg-

* Up to 55 percent of women with symptomatic fibroids have anemia, and another 10 percent have required a blood transfusion at some point due to heavy bleeding.

nancy, fibroids can cause fetal growth restriction, early rupture of membranes (premature water breaking), and preterm birth. Perhaps it's not surprising, then, that in terms of mental health impacts, fibroid diagnoses are also associated with high risks of depression, anxiety, and emotional distress in women over the course of their lives. And so, I understand why some women like Rose would choose to forget about them altogether.

As she continued to pursue her PhD, Rose started noticing clots on top of even heavier bleeding. But she was busy and distracted by the stress of finishing the PhD program. When she graduated and secured a postdoctoral research fellowship across the country, she was ready for a reset. She moved to the West Coast in June of 2018 and remembers long sunny days and endless fresh air. She gave up coffee, changed her eating habits, and lost a good amount of weight in the name of self-care and a fresh start after graduate school. She established new boundaries around work, forgoing internet at home to ensure she could truly disconnect. In this new phase of her life, Rose felt mentally restored and, in many ways, physically healthy.

She had also developed new ways to manage her burdensome periods. She planned her writing days for the times when she would be weakest and bleeding the most to avoid the classroom and meetings. For an academic on the rise, writing up your nascent scientific research is the most critical work you can do, and yet Rose viewed this as less taxing, better suited for the days she would be most physically compromised and needed to stay home. She traveled a great deal for presentations and growing her professional STEM education network. Living in California meant getting anywhere was a long flight. Unlike most frequent flyers who want to conserve time, Rose would purposefully book flights with layovers to ensure shorter plane trips and avoid bleeding accidents. She had begun wearing adult diapers on flights to absorb her blood. Another significant symptom appeared around this time: urinary incontinence. She had pelvic pressure and would leak sometimes, leading her to wear pads even when she wasn't menstruating.

As she recites the details of her endurance and adaptability, she again notes how grateful she was that her cycle was regular. "It meant I could always plan {and} figure out how to manage it," she says. Also, the memories of her high school friends vomiting and laid out on the floor for days loomed large. She'd never been as bad off as they were, she told herself. Her fibroid diagnosis and that little piece of paper on which that doctor had written treatment options remained out of mind. What was happening to her cycles, to her womb, remained compartmentalized and omitted from this otherwise healthy new life. "It was abstract," she says. "I never connected to it as a part of me." As I listen, the disassociation sounds familiar.

Rose was wise to hold on to that paper from her gynecology appointment. But it is likely the case that neither that doctor nor the nurse went into enough detail about her options for Rose to feel empowered to make a well-informed decision about next steps and understand what warning signs should lead her to seek treatment. I am a trained gynecologist, and even I am overwhelmed by fibroid treatment options. Treatment is complicated by the fact that fibroids are caused by different reasons in different people.*

Based on how fibroids impact the body and people's lives, the focus of treatment is: 1) reducing size, 2) controlling abnormal uterine bleeding, and 3) decreasing the risk that they come back. The principles we should use to evaluate the different treatments include whether the patient wants the option to someday carry a pregnancy, whether they have some other reason to keep their uterus, the treatment's expected effectiveness based on the fibroids' specific character-

* For some, epigenetic inheritance and spontaneous mutations cause the uterine stem cells to acquire errors. For others, a gene mutation keeps the myocytes from expressing what they should and makes them act in ways they shouldn't. In still others, alternate gene-protein pathways have a special bonus of messing with the anticoagulation system in the blood, thus promoting longer and heavier periods. There is a different gene region that should decrease cell proliferation but gets turned off (instead of on) by progesterone. The trick with fibroid treatment is finding a way to turn off some of these signals in enough fibroid cells to see a real difference in the growth and disruption they create.

istics, and any risks a patient might have related to procedures or side effects to medications. Depending on those answers, we'll know whether the best approach will be medication, a procedure, or surgery, or a combination.

SUPPLEMENTS FOR FIBROIDS

I promised a discussion of vitamin D for treatment of fibroids, and here it is, along with a few other options. The reason why I believe vitamin D is important is because of how consistent the data is. Generally, nutritional studies are all over the place—one study finds a connection, another one doesn't. Results show up in this population, but don't show up in that one. For vitamin D and fibroids, the connection is consistent across studies and across populations. Now, in general, observing an association (low vitamin D = more fibroids) doesn't mean that one thing causes the other or that you can act to change it. But with this relationship, there are studies that now show that, when women are given vitamin D, fibroid growth stabilizes. There is *not* strong evidence that vitamin D *shrinks* already present fibroids. But it does seem to consistently *halt growth* in a measurable, meaningful way.* Though the data is less strong and less compelling, there is also some clinical evidence that *epigallocatechin (EGCG),* a substance found in green tea, may have some fibroid-stabilization properties as well. When given in combination with vitamin D and vitamin B_6, this therapy showed decreased fibroid size. This data, along with the dietary information from the Black Women's Health Study, make the following recommendations a reasonable and evidence-based approach to any holistic fibroid care plan:

- Eat at least five fruit/vegetable servings per day.
- Limit (or eliminate) fish intake.

* To my physician colleagues, I know that so many of our hopes of vitamin D in other areas of medicine and cancer have been dashed. The large randomized trials have largely failed to show benefit. I would encourage you to check out the fibroid literature. It is promising, and I am hopeful.

- Participate in vigorous exercise or activity for at least > 2hrs/week (at any body size).
- Take vitamin D supplementation to get levels to at least 20 ng/mL.*
- Eliminate chronic stress, leave abusive relationships, and learn to acknowledge, process, and release anger.
- Drinking green tea or taking EGCG supplements may be helpful.

In addition to these efforts, there are many medications and procedures that are effective.

MEDICATIONS FOR FIBROIDS

Medications are primarily used to *decrease abnormal fibroid bleeding*. As you may remember from "Heavy Menstrual Bleeding" (chapter 4) and "Endometriosis" (chapter 5), the goal with medication taken for those conditions is to decrease the amount of endometrial growth. Medications that thin the endometrium so there is less to shed (i.e., combined estrogen and progesterone medication) or improve the clotting functions (i.e., tranexamic acid) combat fibroid bleeding too. NSAIDs, most commonly in the form of ibuprofen, naproxen, or diclofenac, are also a godsend for fibroids, as they lower the inflammatory prostaglandins that fan the flames of bleeding and pain. Progesterone-containing IUDs can be helpful, though with fibroids these can have a higher expulsion rate *if* fibroids are large enough to distort the uterine cavity's shape. That can make it difficult for the IUD to stay put. These approaches are great options for fibroids that are worsening bleeding but are not too large or causing severe pressure symptoms.

Some medications also help directly by *decreasing fibroid size*. GnRH (gonadotropin-releasing hormone) agonists and antagonists

* From the research, the recommended dosing is 50,000 IU weekly for eight weeks, then 2,000 IU per day. Patients with larger bodies may need higher doses. I say "at least 20 ng/mL" because studies of women with vitamin D above this level still demonstrated benefit of additional vitamin D.

are strong hormonal medications that stop the brain and ovaries from working together to create estrogen and other sex steroid hormones. Fibroid cells need the signal from estrogen to use progesterone to keep growing, so shutting down their communication significantly stifles fibroid growth. One of the most common GnRH agonists is leuprolide acetate. Ninety-eight percent of women who use it stop excessive bleeding completely, and it also makes fibroids on average 35–65 percent smaller. That can mean a fibroid that has been pressing on your bladder such that you need to go to the bathroom four times an hour shrinks and leaves your bladder alone.

There is a catch. The menopausal side effects of GnRH agonists like leuprolide acetate are significant, and if they are taken for longer than six months, bone loss can become a problem, so they are temporary medications only. For this reason, people on these medications will also sometimes take a small amount of progesterone (in the form of norethindrone acetate) that can help relieve the menopausal symptoms without re-triggering fibroid growth. This is called *add-back therapy*. Fibroids will regrow after a few months of stopping these medications. Thus, they are not long-term solutions, but they have an important role in treatment. They are used presurgery or preprocedure to shrink fibroids and improve anemia, which can allow someone to have a minimally invasive surgery rather than a large abdominal incision. These are important to discuss with any surgeon suggesting a procedure as a way to reduce risk.

In addition, there are oral GnRH antagonists, such as elagolix and relugolix. These are pills that work in a similar way to leuprolide acetate, but they can be used much longer, for up to two years. They have a longer use because they come in a combined form with an estrogen and progesterone, so they do not deplete hormone levels to the degree that the GnRH agonist (leuprolide acetate) would.* They can also stabilize fibroid size while they are taken—an excellent option when, for example, you need something to stop and stabilize growth, while taking time to consider if surgery is right for you.

* At the time of writing, the common commercial names for these combined pills are Oriahnn and Myfembree.

As I've mentioned, the ovaries aren't the only places that produce estrogen. Fat cells, skin cells, and other areas do also, often through the *aromatase* enzyme. Aromatase inhibitors (AIs) are medications that target these other estrogen producers and can bring about a 40–50 percent reduction in fibroid size. Women of African descent express more aromatase, and thus this treatment could be even more effective among us. And here is a caveat: Aromatase inhibitors to treat fibroids are what we call an "off-label" use for this medication. This means that they were not developed to treat fibroids specifically, but clinicians have noticed, and it has been backed up by research, that they do affect fibroids. When a medication is used off-label, it may not be available to everyone due to insurance limitations or simply being inappropriate given other patient factors to consider.

Selective progesterone receptor modulators (SPRMs, which we call "sperms" for short) block progesterone receptors, which directly inhibit the growth of fibroids and thin the endometrium. SPRMs, which are sometimes also called *anti-progestins,* shrink fibroids in half and control over 90 percent of excessive bleeding. They can be used preoperatively in the same way as GnRH agonists or in short, three-month bursts for someone not planning on surgery. The most common SPRM is called ulipristal acetate. It has been studied the most, is the safest, and works well without the menopausal symptoms that make the GnRH agonists difficult to take. And yet, this medication is highly regulated, difficult to obtain, and deeply understocked by most pharmacies. Ostensibly, the reason for this is a rare but severe possibility of liver toxicity. But it's also the case that ulipristal, like all SPRMs, blocks progesterone in the uterus, and so prevents a newly joined egg and sperm from implanting on the uterine wall, the first step to establish a pregnancy. In the United States, it goes by another label: the morning-after pill. Our governments and lawmakers are so focused on incorrectly stigmatizing this drug as only an abortion pill that they prioritize its restriction over the potential benefit of millions of women with fibroids who could use it to improve their quality of life, relieve symptoms, and avoid surgeries. No one aspect of gynecologic or reproductive care exists in a silo. Banning abortion means banning our access to the full range of gynecologic healthcare, period.

PROCEDURES FOR FIBROIDS

I will refer to a treatment approach as a *procedure* rather than *surgery* when the clinician is neither cutting into the patient nor removing anything. But procedures *are* invasive. They require direct access to the inside of the body and use something external to induce fibroid shrinkage and resolution. Procedures work, until they don't. They can be an ideal option for people who want to keep their uterus, who don't mind ultimately needing repeat procedures, and who are not interested in carrying any future pregnancies.

Uterine artery embolization (UAE) shrinks fibroids by depriving them of blood, which they need to survive and grow. The doctor introduces gelatin microspheres or polyvinyl alcohol into the small blood vessels that feed the target fibroid. This immediately stops growth, then causes the fibroid cells to die off. Four in ten women will experience fibroid shrinkage, shorter periods, and improvement in bulk symptoms after this procedure. In a large study of over 1,300 women, Black women had a notably high rate of choosing UAE. One in five Black women chose this procedure compared to just 7–8 percent of other races. These women reported improvements in quality of life, bleeding, bulk/pressure, and pain at one year out equal to others who had surgeries. But for some the effect from UAE faded by three years out. Within five years, about 20 percent of women who have this procedure will need another to address their fibroids.

Radiofrequency ablation (RF) is a procedure that treats fibroids by applying radiofrequency energy to the fibroid directly, causing the cells to die off. This makes the fibroid shrink significantly. There are two ways to enter the uterus to get to the fibroids—either through the cervix (transcervical) or through the surface of the uterus (laparoscopic). RF is an outpatient procedure done in the office or an ambulatory surgical center. It's gaining in popularity both in the United States and internationally as an alternative to UAE. Three months after an RF ablation, fibroid size shrinks by at least 40 percent, on average. In one of the largest trials following participants' outcomes for years, only 11 percent of women needed another RF intervention for their fibroids after five years.

Magnetic resonance (MR) guided focused ultrasound is a much rarer but also effective procedure. It uses an MRI and high-frequency ultrasound waves to induce the blood clotting in fibroid tissue, killing the fibroid cells and shrinking the tumors. It has important limitations and is best on people with fewer than five fibroids and none larger than 10 cm, among other considerations. Over 70 percent of women who get this procedure report improvement of symptoms at six months, but one in three (33 percent) will need another procedure or surgery eventually.

The final procedure to cover is *endometrial ablation,* which is the burning and scarring of the endometrial lining. This is different from the MRI-based ablation above, since it does not shrink or treat the fibroids themselves, but targets only the bleeding.* Between 29 and 40 percent of people who choose ablation have recurring symptoms or eventually have another operation. Endometrial ablation fails most commonly among people with larger fibroids, who are forty-five or older, and who also have severely painful periods or severe adenomyosis, a gynecologic condition where endometrial tissue grows in the muscle layer of the uterus. I am not a big fan of endometrial ablation. I believe it's a Band-Aid rather than a direct treatment and does not do anything to slow or prevent fibroid growth. It's something, though, and Rose, years out from her only gynecology visit, had nothing.

In the early days of the pandemic, Rose began having difficulty breathing, especially at night. She was worried she had COVID, but the advice at that time was to stay away from hospitals unless one's symptoms were truly unbearable. She drank chai tea to stay awake when her breathing was especially labored and called family mem-

* See chapter 4, "Heavy Menstrual Bleeding," for detailed discussion of this treatment.

bers to sit up with her on FaceTime. Over a telehealth visit, her assigned primary care doctor suggested she may have acid reflux and prescribed her an antacid for relief. He did not ask about her gynecologic health. Her breathing did not get better. She relied on Google searches to answer her many questions: Could she have sleep apnea? Could she get a sleep study in the middle of lockdown? She couldn't, but she was able to get in to see an ear, nose, and throat specialist. After an exam, she was reassured nothing was wrong. "Everyone was telling me everything was looking normal, but I did not feel normal."

Soon, the Black Lives Matter movement disrupted life in new ways. At her university, the frenzy for institutional anti-racist work was affecting every Black faculty member. Rose, a physical chemist, a gifted science educator, and a Black woman with a passion for mentoring and leadership, answered the call. She founded a mentoring program almost overnight and began convening Black STEM panels on campus. She also started a mentorship group of Black undergraduate and graduate students and was seemingly a part of every discussion on how to address the chronic shortage of Black scholars in scientific disciplines.

I met Rose when she asked me to be on one of her panels on this topic. We had connected through social media. I immediately agreed. I remember being in awe of her during these years. She seemed to be everywhere at once, constantly creating quality programming for her mentoring program and others across campuses. I know now that she was also still bleeding, a lot. I asked how this was possible. "I don't think I was paying attention . . . to what was happening with my body," she tells me. "My mentoring program kept me so focused. I'm getting things done. My period comes, I'm knocked out. I do the ibuprofen schedule, sleep, my energy pops back up, I'm good."

Eventually, she would realize she was not "good." She had upgraded her bleeding management and was now using diapers not only for flights but for every monthly cycle. The clots went from annoying to alarming. "They got heavier and heavier. They were big, extremely big. I had never seen anything like that in my life. This is not normal. Like, it didn't feel human, Kemi." She googled to see how much blood was a normal amount to lose in a cycle and was shocked. "This can't be for Black women," she remembers thinking. "I've never in my life had the volume they are describing." She was now straining all her strategies, using the doubled-up pads in addition to diapers, not leaving the house on cycle days, avoiding people and meetings due to weakness. The clots continued, and they began to seem too big and too thick to even just be blood alone. Rose called her mother, genuinely concerned she was dying. And, finally, at the point of maxing out all other strategies, she told her primary care doctor. He ordered an ultrasound.

By then, it had been about three years since that first ultrasound in graduate school when Rose learned of her fibroids, heard the word *centimeters,* and so assumed they were insignificant. It had been three years since she received that piece of paper with her three options. For the first time since then, she wondered how her fibroids connected to what was going on with her cycle and with her breathing. During her ultrasound, it took a while for the technician to capture all the images, because her fibroids were so big. She remembers the technician saying "Whoa," and struggling to get the right angles. When Rose's doctor called her with the results, the tenor of the conversation had changed: "You have fibroids, they are big, and you need to see a surgeon." Rose immediately went into problem-solving mode. She remembered me from the panels and scheduled an appointment, happy to travel for care.

We ordered a battery of tests, and Rose felt relieved that she had data to look at. Her scientist self could latch on to the lab work and to the additional imaging studies. A CT scan showed her uterus was completely distended with fibroids. She now had information that showed, given the size and location of her fibroids, a *myomectomy,* or targeted surgical approach, would be insufficient. She remembers when I drew her a picture of the uterus, then compared normal anatomy to what we were seeing on her scans. That's the first time it clicked, she tells me now. "I'm still thinking at this point, it's the reflux, it's other things. Maybe y'all don't know I have a weird type of COVID, anything . . . until you made that drawing." That day, I had to tell Rose that the options her doctor had written on that paper years before were no longer options. Her fibroids were larger and had taken over too much of her normal uterine architecture to make less invasive and less permanent treatments viable options. The fibroids pressed on her diaphragm and crowded her lungs, which, along with her anemia, was why she was struggling with breathing. She asked me to be honest with her about what treatment would be most effective, and I was: She needed a hysterectomy.

What we are taught in medical school, or sometimes what I think of as the "fairy-tale" story of fibroids, goes like this: Fibroids usually grow in the years when women have active menstrual cycles and regress, or shrink down, after menopause. If you happen to have fibroids, you just need to outlast them to menopause, and you'll be okay because they will disappear—or at least shrink so much they are barely noticed. Up to a quarter of fibroids (23 percent) will appear, grow rapidly up to 2 cm, and then spontaneously shrink. They are short-lived, showing up and disappearing within a couple of years. Smaller fibroids are most likely to quickly regress. And then, as women age into perimenopause and beyond, all fibroids—regardless of size—tend to regress as well. That is the fairy tale. The reality for Black women is different. Epidemiologist Dr. Donna Baird followed nearly 1,700 young Black women to track new fibroids and fibroid growth. Among her participants who had never had a fibroid diagnosis and did not believe they had fibroids, 21 percent (one in five) of them actually already did. For those who were truly fibroid-free, 9 percent developed their first fibroid over the year-and-a-half-long observation period.* They were able to truly track fibroid growth in this study. It took a 2 cm fibroid about four to five years to double in size, and once a fibroid reached 4 cm, it was *much* less likely to go away on its own. From other studies, we also know that for Black women, the expected fibroid regression in older women is slower if it happens at

* This was not a study where anyone was given anything. The researchers just followed along, doing ultrasounds to check for fibroids as the women lived their usual lives.

all. What this means is that Black women, especially in their twenties and thirties, are more likely to be struggling with more symptomatic, larger, and more persistent fibroids than anyone else. Rose was one of those women.

"I couldn't believe it's been just three, four years, whatever the time difference, from 'you don't have to worry about this right now' to here," she says. After meeting with me for a consultation, Rose went full speed ahead to "fix" her fibroids. While she is recalling this period of her life to me, she admits she couldn't really process the impact of surgery and what it meant for her as someone who had not yet had any children at the time. She had a second preoperative visit with my colleague, another gynecologic oncologist and surgeon, to review the paperwork ahead of surgery. She spoke to a friend who'd had a hysterectomy and who was very encouraging to Rose, extolling the benefits and how she would feel "so much lighter." She looked briefly into egg freezing and decided to take our recommendation of preserving her ovaries in her body and not removing them. She was overwhelmed, though she says a few times, she didn't really feel pressured by us, just pressured to "solve this problem."* She kept thinking, *How did I, like, miss all of this?* She had understood that one day she would need to deal with her fibroids, but she felt caught off guard. "I didn't think I would need something so soon."

Rose had a hysterectomy on February 2, 2021. Her uterus and all its fibroids were removed. She kept her ovaries. She could breathe again. She stopped taking iron. Two days after she was discharged from the hospital, she submitted another research grant. She said her postoperative instructions didn't include anything about "not using my brain." That's just the way she's wired.

---

* In listening back to our interview, I realized I asked this question in about five different ways, the repetition exposing my worry that I had, in my enthusiasm to help her feel better as her doctor, inappropriately pressured Rose in this vulnerable time. She told me no, repeatedly, but honestly, I still worry.

SURGICAL TREATMENT FOR FIBROIDS

The two major surgeries for fibroid treatment are *myomectomy* and *hysterectomy*. They make up over 90 percent of all invasive fibroid treatment. These options remove the fibroid itself, rather than relying on medicine or a procedure to shrink it. A myomectomy is the removal of a single or multiple fibroids while preserving the uterus. In the case of myomectomy, the direct removal of fibroids increases the chance that the individual fibroid stem cells, which started the whole process of growth, are removed as well. The way a myomectomy is done depends on the location and size of the fibroids. When fibroids are within or very close to the *endometrium,* they can be resected from inside the uterus using a small camera and instruments inserted through the cervix. This is called a *hysteroscopic myomectomy* and is an outpatient procedure that leaves no surgical scars.

When fibroids are in the middle muscle layer (myometrium) or outer layer (serosa) of the uterus, they are removed through an incision made in the abdominal wall. Depending on the size and location of the fibroids as well as on the skill and training of the surgeon, these fibroids can be removed via minimally invasive small incisions or a single large incision. Myomectomy is ideal when future fertility (via one's own womb, as opposed to surrogacy) is desired or there is a desire to keep one's uterus, regardless of reproductive plans. This surgical approach reduces symptoms 80 percent of the time, with nearly 75 percent of women who only needed a single fibroid removed not needing further treatment. For those needing multiple fibroids removed, about half will not need further treatment.

A hysterectomy, the removal of the uterus, is what we in gynecology call the definitive treatment for fibroids. It does *not* include the removal of the ovaries and does *not* result in menopause. With a hysterectomy, the chance of fibroid symptoms returning or of one needing another procedure is essentially 0 percent. Removing the uterus means there are no more fibroids and no more fibroid stem cells to grow them. When comparing fibroid treatments, quality-of-life data favors hysterectomy because it is the only treatment that stops 100 percent of all bleeding, so even if pain symptoms persist, hysterectomy often still results in reduced symptoms overall. Similar to myomectomy, there are three different approaches to hysterectomy: vaginal, a minimally invasive approach using laparoscopic or robotic instruments, and an abdominal incision. Though it is a larger surgery, the major complication rate is low at 0.4 percent. As I've mentioned, fewer than half a percent of all fibroids are cancerous. But when cancer is discovered, hysterectomy is also the only treatment that would remove potentially cancerous cells safely.

More than 99 percent of fibroids are noncancerous, but every so often, that is not the case. When I was in my fellowship training in 2015, I met a fellow ob-gyn who was a new patient of one of my supervising doctors. She came in knowing she wanted a hysterectomy, as her fibroids were large, growing, and too uncomfortable for her to continue managing them as she had been. She was in her mid-forties, and she knew what all of us gynecologists did: Fibroids were incredibly common among Black women, who were less likely to see the regression and symptom relief typically associated with menopause. So, we counseled her that although new fibroid growth could be a sign of malignancy, it was exceedingly rare (less than 1 percent of all fibroid surgeries result in discovery of a cancerous fibroid). We would be prepared to adjust the surgery as needed if further investigation showed cancer was a risk. As gynecologic oncologists, we could do surgery for both benign and cancerous growths. She understood. This was part of the reason she had chosen our team, and she was eager to have her hysterectomy and start feeling better.

When we opened her up, we found that her fibroids were indeed cancerous—*leiomyosarcoma,* to be specific. She was a slight woman, and I remember wondering how she was even eating and keeping food down considering how extensively her bowels were compressed and shoved aside by her large, cancerous uterus. The surgery itself went smoothly. I don't remember much about her initial stay in the hospital after her surgery, other than realizing, with a bit of a startle, that we kind of looked alike. (A medical student pointed this out, and then I couldn't unsee it.) We had a similar rich brown skin tone, short natural hair, and even the same style of glasses. Most of the patients we cared for were in their sixties and up, and I saw and treated them as respected elders. But this patient was, like me, a Black woman ob-gyn and also closer in age to me, perhaps a decade older at most. I focused on being competent and respectful and on engaging her as a colleague. We exchanged warm smiles each morning as she recovered. I recognized her consistent composure and her focus on immediate next steps as similar to how I would respond to unexpected challenges. She went home a few days after surgery to heal.

It wasn't long before she was back. I was making rounds in the hospital at the time but was called down to clinic by my attending, her doctor, to see her. She was struggling with constipation and abdominal pain at home and couldn't manage anymore. "Let's bring her in and get her teed up, Kemi. I think some hydration, bowel rest, and good pain medications can get her turned around again," my supervisor said. I agreed. I chatted with the patient a bit in the exam room, reassured her that relief was coming, as I saw the fatigue and strain on her face, and got my team activated to admit her once again to our inpatient ward.

As part of a routine step, we ordered imaging to ensure there was no issue from the surgery, such as scar tissue or infection, that may have been causing a mechanical bowel blockage. I clicked open her electronic chart, and my heart sank at the results. There was no scar tissue or infection. It was worse. There was cancer. Everywhere. In just a few weeks, the cancer cells were regrowing with abandon. In most cases of solid tumors, the three-to-six-week recovery period is normal before treatment begins, to allow the body to heal. For a cancer to regrow in that amount of time is an extremely poor sign.* I

* No, surgery does not cause cancer to spread. This is an old myth that originated in the days when we didn't have good imaging studies, so folks didn't know how extensive cancer was until a surgery was done. To the patient, the cancer was "just" in her womb and then it was everywhere. What is true is that outside of a few specific scenarios, surgery *alone* does not necessarily stop cancer from coming back, because there may be cancer stem cells still present in the body. This is why many cancers need treatment after surgery to prevent regrowth. This patient's regrowth was concerning because of how *fast* it happened.

hated this news and hated that I had to share it with her. But I did. She had taken the initial news of the leiomyosarcoma diagnosis relatively well. Now, she was devastated. We still had the same goal: get her eating, hydrate her, and ease her pain so she could start treatment. But the outlook was much grimmer.

She never left the hospital. I felt connected to this woman in a way that is hard to describe but that felt like an energetic cord. I sought her out whether I was assigned to the wards or not. I thought about her before I drifted off to sleep and woke up to check her labs and her status each morning. I spoke with her as much as I could, first about her condition, then about anything. She declined quickly. Her parents came to be with her. When I helped her transition to a Do Not Resuscitate (DNR) status, I left the room with tears rolling down my face. My team of medical students and resident trainees watched in stunned silence. I worked for years to establish a warm, but distant, authority with them as a rare Black woman in my position. No matter how stressful our long days were, I did not cry in front of them. Ever. But this patient cracked through my armor. I continued to care for her. I noticed her mother steadfastly avoided looking at my face. I could understand why. Her father was the opposite. I held his gaze when she could no longer make eye contact. He hugged me when he could no longer hug her.

At the time, I thought she had just the worst kind of luck. Now I understand her case differently. When she came to us, her uterus, huge and filled with fibroids, pressed against her other organs. She was fatigued and couldn't fit into her regular clothes. Now I wonder if she had sought help sooner, would we have been able to save her? I wonder about the very first time she noticed something was off. When did she find out she had fibroids? When was the first time she noticed pressure on her bladder? What crossed her mind when she went to put on a pair of pants and they didn't fit, so she switched to one with a stretchier waist? Had her desire to have children led her to wait to seek treatment? Why do we live in a society where a breast mass has women running to the doctor but a growing fibroid uterus is more often accommodated? How had she managed to work and learn in a field that routinely communicates, *Yes, Black women dispro-*

portionately suffer from fibroids, shrug, *we don't really know why?* She was an ob-gyn. She knew the truth about large fibroids: We had little to offer her other than surgery. I can't fault her logic when what she learned professionally and from society was that how we deal with fibroids can be summed up by one word: *neglect.*

~

Rose's hysterectomy had led to a more positive outcome, but as we talk now several years later, she is still wrestling with her decision and grieving her fertility. She tells me she used to joke that she would always choose a surrogate to bear children, because she had no interest in the pain of childbirth. Surrogacy is still an option for her, but now that path feels different. She is partly happy she doesn't have to fear childbirth as a Black woman in the United States, where maternal morbidity and mortality are a real threat. But she has suffered a loss. One she is still actively mourning. "I remember when I first found out about fibroids, I just did a little research. I knew sometimes they shrink and sometimes they can block the birth canal if you are pregnant. So, I was thinking that I had to be aware of that when the time came for me to have a baby. But otherwise, I'm just moving on to the next step of my life. I'm just not thinking about them every day. It just wasn't connected to what I was going through, in my mind." Except for her mother, she also hasn't told anyone about her surgery. She did not tell her best friend, her brother or father, her godmother, no one. "I just need time," she tells me. For a while, she would ask that this surgical history not be included in her medical record, because "that would make it real." She has recovered physically, but not emotionally or mentally.

The natural light is fading in the room we sit in as the sun sets. She shakes her head, almost bewildered, when thinking about how much she was doing while living through this Womb Suffering. I notice one of her patterns—saying "at least" to convince herself everything was under control. At least she wasn't vomiting. At least her cycles were regular. At least when she needed surgery, she felt she had the best team in the world. "A lot of people are badly advised, Kemi," she tells me. "At least I had that." She also lights up when she talks about the legacy of the mentoring program. Her mentee, a Black woman who recently obtained her undergraduate degree, wasn't sure if she could be successful in medical school. She was accepted to not one but three MD-PhD programs. Rose is proud when she notes how many similar stories she has accumulated. "I don't want to get to a place where I wonder if what happened would have been different if I wasn't doing all of that institutional work, you know? But if I didn't do the work, would I have clocked what was going on? Would I have been able to choose one of those other options?"

As we wrap up, I ask Rose where she thinks she learned to keep going as long as her symptoms were "manageable." "I think that's just what's expected of us," she said. "All the women in my life do it. We all do it." She mentioned a kind of mantra that's often repeated among Black people, expression of a shared belief that our efforts must outpace those of White people to get even a sliver of the recognition they receive. " 'You gotta work twice as hard.' That's just what society expects." But that's not the message she gives to others now. "Whenever I hear a friend mentioning something not going well down there or having fibroids, I'm like, 'You have to go see someone *now*.' " Though many in her circle still do not know of her surgery, Rose is committed to helping them avoid her fate, if possible. Rose has also noticed a greater dialogue about gynecologic health in recent years. The social media posts, often prompted by a terrible story of medical neglect, have prompted a different kind of "me too" in the comments from women similarly suffering in silence. "I don't think I had a real womb discussion until my visit [for my hysterectomy]." At eight years old, she was taught about teen pregnancy. Then she was taught how to use pads. "And not anything else," she concludes.

But I think Rose *was* taught many other things, indirectly. She was taught that her womb was only for getting pregnant and that it would bleed every month. She was taught that if she wasn't completely physically incapacitated, then nothing was wrong. She was taught to ignore it until she finished her studies, got married, and was ready to have a baby. She was taught that when she seeks care for her womb, she needs to be on guard because she can't trust the motivations of her doctors. She was taught that as long as she can manage, she should. She came from the top girls school in her country, where everyone was taught to succeed. And she put pursuing that success first.

"I think we've all just settled in where someone says, 'Oh, it's just pain. Just go take something. Go take that green pill,'" she told me. "We've just figured out a way as women, how to deal with it. So, no one cares. And if we die, it's, 'It's just one {woman}. It's not everybody.'"

Neglect, disassociation, and distancing from a fibroid diagnosis are rational responses to the current state of knowledge and treatment options for fibroids. It also makes sense for Black women to respond in these ways given the risks we face when pursuing gynecologic health. We are less likely to have our pain be believed, we are more likely to experience coercion toward birth control methods we don't want, and we are less likely to experience a quality, respectful conversation with our doctors. Fibroids are hidden, their damage is rarely fatal, and you can forget about them. In learning how to neglect my own needs on my path to success, I gained the skills I used to neglect the growing fibroid in my uterus. But misplaced strength and self-neglect are destroying Black women's quality of life. These tools work to get us through the day, but not toward the thriving lives we deserve. Living this way is a hard habit to break, despite all the other hard-won wisdom we accumulate. As we get older, so do our wombs—and the signs that something is off get quieter, subtler, and can be the difference between life and death. This is the world that increasingly faces our matriarchs. The threat they face—endometrial cancer—is where we will take our last womb journey.

CHAPTER 7

ENDOMETRIAL CANCER

The Deadly Womb

Cancer is fundamentally a disease of imbalance. The natural order of our cells is to emerge, grow, function, and die. We are a system of trillions of cells that are in one of those four stages at any given time. Different kinds of cells move through those stages at different speeds—some have the lifespan of a day, others decades. Regardless, they all share one critical job—to die off when they no longer function correctly. With cancer, those cells don't die. Instead, they malfunction and keep growing.

Internally, our bodies have a first line of defense. If a malfunctioning cell doesn't self-destruct, our immune system sends wonderful hunting cells that go on the offensive. With cancer, this system fails. These hunting cells sail right on by, tricked by how "normal" the malfunctioning cells look on the outside. Outside of the body, we have two more lines of defense—first, the troubling symptoms that send us to the doctor for help, and then, finally, treatments to help our bodies remove these cells. With endometrial cancer, the checks and balances fail at multiple points, creating cascading and often fatal consequences.

Endometrial, or uterine, cancer is the most common gynecologic cancer diagnosed in the United States, yet we almost never hear it discussed in the media or in our friendship circles. It is three times as common as ovarian cancer and five times more common than cervical cancer, yet many women who have the disease will say something like "I had never heard of this until I was diagnosed." There are more endometrial cancer than colon cancer cases in the US. By 2050, it will be more common than lung cancer—making it the second-most-common cancer in the United States after breast cancer for anyone with a uterus.

Endometrial cancer is not a new disease. Since the mid-1970s when a national cancer surveillance network was launched in the United States, we have been tracking these uterine cancer rates. We have numbers on both *incidence rates,* or how commonly it occurs, and *mortality rates*, or how many folks who get it die within five years. For decades, there have been two consistent facts about endometrial cancer: 1) Most White women get low-risk, nonaggressive endometrial cancer generally curable through hysterectomy, and 2) Black women more often get high-risk, aggressive endometrial cancer that requires significant treatment after surgery and is responsible for most endometrial cancer deaths. This was true in 1980, and it is true today. What's changed is that today endometrial cancer is more common for everyone.* The survival difference between Black and White women, however, has only gotten worse.

With endometrial cancer, the womb nurtures a cancer instead of a new life. It is a cancer that most often strikes when a woman is finished with her reproductive years. The average age of diagnosis is sixty-three years old, and endometrial cancer becomes the final chapter of a gynecologic life story. Black women have more than double

* Endometrial cancer follows the pattern of many health disparities for other racial and ethnic groups. Aggressive types are more common among Latinas (32 percent), Asian / Pacific Islanders (34 percent), and Native Americans (32 percent) compared to White women (30 percent). And within Latinas, rates vary by race: 32 percent for White Latinas compared to 48 percent for Black Latinas. When we see these patterns following the way we know the social desirability ladder works in the United States, we know the problem is not genetic—it's societal.

the chance of death after a diagnosis of endometrial cancer than White women. That's over 100 percent higher risk. (For context, in breast cancer, the increased risk for Black women is 38 percent.) These are the odds I knew each one of my Black patients with endometrial cancer was up against when I treated them. The very first such woman in my care was Ms. Barbara Collins.

When I greet Ms. Barbara at my door in October of 2024, she is wearing a classic white sweatsuit, and short gray locs adorn her head. It's been about a year since I last saw her, and this is her first time at my home. I was nervous when I reached out to see if she would allow me to share her story. Ms. Barbara is a grandmother of three who owns a thriving restaurant in the revitalized Seattle Central District. In 2017, she entrusted her life to me and went under my knife. Any oncologist will tell you that for how many patients we lose and have to say goodbye to, there are always just enough wins to keep going. Ms. Barbara was a win for me. I am beaming as she gingerly makes it down the steps to my front door, as I'm feeling immense gratitude for her survival and her willingness to speak with me. She crosses the threshold and envelops me in a tight hug. "I'm so honored. I'm so grateful. I'm so glad to see you," she tells me. After getting her settled in my family's living room and triple-checking my two recording devices, I calm my nerves and we begin.

Ms. Barbara was born and raised in West Point, Mississippi, a small town where her family were sharecroppers who picked cotton. Her mother, Rev. Mary Elizabeth Hammond, had Barbara as a teenager and worked from sunup to sundown, she tells me. She worked all day in a café and always had a side hustle. Rev. Mary was a beautician on the weekends, made pies for the community, transformed her small home into a boardinghouse for girls, and even ran a restaurant at one point. And she always had time for her daughter.

"We were more like sisters than mother and daughter," Ms. Barbara remembers. Despite evidence of their close relationship, when I ask how she learned about menstruation, her mother is not part of the story. "Oh, we did not talk about down there," she says and tells me this would have been a shameful topic to bring up. Instead, Ms. Barbara smiles as she talks about learning from a "cool" schoolteacher from Chicago. When Ms. Barbara started her period around twelve years old, it was this teacher who taught her how to use pads, follow a calendar to prepare herself, and generally maintain her cleanliness. When she was sixteen, Ms. Barbara met an older man, who was twenty-one, and got pregnant quickly. At that time in small-town Mississippi, getting pregnant meant getting married, and so they did. Ms. Barbara would be married to him for twenty years and have two more children. She never mentions his name, and I do not ask. Her retelling hints at a kind of terror I don't want to ask her to relive. He impregnated her when he was an adult and she was a child. He cheated on her repeatedly and had at least one child outside of the marriage.

Like many other Black families, Ms. Barbara left the Deep South in the 1960s. Along with her husband and children, her mother and her mother's sister, she relocated to Washington State for a better life. Ms. Barbara worked her day job at Kaiser Permanente, sold Mary Kay on the weekends, and took any other odd job that paid. "I'm going to do my thing and get my money," she says, remembering those days with a chuckle. Many women simply can't leave their abusive and controlling marriages, but Ms. Barbara did. After twenty years of saving enough, she packed up one day and left while he was out of the house, moving across the state to Seattle with her daughters. She did not tell a soul where she went, including her mother. For months, she was free.

"I was partying one night, just having a good old time," she tells me. "I walked out of the club and somebody grabs me, and it was him. He was talking about what he was gonna do. He was going to kill me and all that. I said, 'Well, you know, at this point, I don't really care.'" She tells me how in that moment her own survival didn't feel important, but she urged her husband to consider what their daughters would think of him. She knew that despite his many failures, he loved those girls. He forced her into his car and drove her to her Seattle home in silence. She didn't see him again for decades.*

* Ms. Barbara was lucky. The highest risk of death is when someone leaves an abusive relationship. If you are in a controlling relationship and fear for your safety, call

I have conducted research interviews with Black women from all walks of life and from every corner of the United States for over a decade now. I am no longer surprised when, in a matter-of-fact manner, they recount traumatic experiences that might derail others for the rest of their lives. When Black women stoically recount the atrocities they've endured, it enrages me. I know the lack of emotion in their voices is born of the strength they have had to carry. So today, as Ms. Barbara recounts this life-threatening experience casually, I just release a deep and heavy sigh.

Ms. Barbara kept living her life. In the 1990s, she began working at Costco, quickly rising through their ranks to become a store manager. She raised her daughters and did her best to teach them what she hadn't been taught so they could avoid early pregnancies and terrible marriages. In 2011, her oldest daughter, now an adult, encouraged Ms. Barbara to sell the delicious pies that she was known for. Her Costco co-workers also urged her to give it a go. She decided to try selling her pies at a local Saturday farmers market. On a Friday night after work, Ms. Barbara stayed up past four o'clock in the morning making one hundred pies in a local commissary kitchen. Hours later, she sold all one hundred pies in ninety minutes. "Everyone else at the market is still working, and we're sold out," she tells me, beaming with pride. "We went to a café, put our feet up, and just watched the market for the rest of the day." A few years later, she opened Simply Soulful, a bakery turned restaurant that sells her sweet potato pies and several other soul food dishes. She kept her "good job" at Costco, spent many late nights in the commissary kitchen, and enlisted her daughter to help out in the café. In 2015, Simply Soulful got a write-up in our local newspaper, *The Seattle Times,* and business boomed.

As we talk, Ms. Barbara mentions major health conditions that are seemingly footnotes in her story. While stocking at Costco in her forties, she noticed it was increasingly hard to breathe and she was

the US National Domestic Violence Hotline at 800-799-7233, text 88788, or visit TheHotline.org for resources and to set up a strong safety plan to best protect yourself to leave.

diagnosed with heart failure from a valve tear. She was placed on medication to improve the symptoms and was grateful she didn't need surgery, which would have required time off work. Over the years, she developed thyroid disease, atrial fibrillation, and hypertension. She faithfully went to all her doctors' appointments and took her medications to manage all these conditions. She kept working. In fact, Ms. Barbara is what I was taught to think of in medical school as a "model patient." She did her Pap smear and mammogram every year. She checked all the healthcare boxes she was supposed to with little complaint. So how did she end up in my office in 2017 with advanced-stage, aggressive endometrial cancer that only one in four women survive?

Through 2020, endometrial cancer research was barely funded by the National Cancer Institute. The CDC's first public health campaign that actually included endometrial cancer was not until 2007.* Endometrial cancer was, to our US cancer community and public health system, simply not a priority problem. I think this is because White women, with a survival rate of over 85 percent, from a population perspective were largely doing fine.†

Things have changed in recent years, and endometrial cancer is beginning to get the attention it deserves from the research and public health communities. I wish I believed this was because of ongoing "racial awakenings" from high-profile police violence in the United States or because the 2020 COVID pandemic has shifted how racial health equity is treated and addressed. Maybe these contributed, but a much larger force is at play. For the first time recorded, White women are starting to get more aggressive endometrial cancers too. For reasons we do not yet understand, they are starting

* The *CDC Inside Knowledge: Get The Facts About Gynecologic Cancer* brochure, page 16. How many of you saw it?

† When I was in training, I was told that endometrial cancer was the "good" cancer to get—if you had to get a gyn cancer. Most women just needed surgery, and most were cured. Black women weren't part of this blithe summary. Their deaths weren't part of the story.

to get them more commonly and they are starting to die in larger numbers.

Cue the interest. Cue the research dollars. Cue the public health awareness.

I can't help but wonder where we would be if we cared about Black women's lives with the same focus and intensity. Where would we be now with addressing endometrial cancer if Black women dropping dead within a year of diagnosis of a cancer that is usually curable was cause for national concern? If it had been Barbara Walters who died within a year of diagnosis instead of the legendary Black journalist Gwen Ifill, would the loss have been met by our health-conscious media with the same relative silence? Would it have still taken years for endometrial cancer to be highlighted in official testimony to Congress by leaders at the NIH?

We've been speaking for an hour, talking in depth about her health, and Ms. Barbara hasn't once mentioned bleeding. So, I ask her directly about her gynecologic health. It turns out her periods were regular and she assumed she was in good gynecologic health because her Pap smears were always negative. This is one of the most common refrains I hear from women who are angry, frustrated, and scared with a new endometrial cancer diagnosis. "But my Pap smears were fine!" They didn't know the Pap is not designed to test for endometrial cancer or that up until very recently, no one thought it important to screen for endometrial cancer symptoms. How would they know? Ms. Barbara tells me that sometime in her mid-sixties her periods became irregular. I collect my thoughts, cycling through ways to delve deeper. Menopause is clinically defined as the cessation of monthly bleeding for at least twelve months and marks the end of menstruation. The average age of menopause in the United States is fifty-one years old, and we expect it to have occurred for nearly everyone by sixty. As menopause approaches, bleeding will get irregular and *lighter*. Though a few heavier or longer cycles as a person gets close to their last bleed are relatively common (about a third of women), these heavier cycles should not last for years. Such a pattern during traditional menopausal years is concerning. I ask Ms. Barbara when she expected her own menopause transition, and she had no idea. "We [she and her mother] didn't talk about that." What about her ob-gyn? Did they ask her about menopausal symptoms or check in on her bleeding patterns? Unfortunately, the answer is no. Ms. Barbara experienced something increasingly common in this country, as reproductive rights are rolled back and women's healthcare becomes scarcer over time. Her ob-gyn closed their gynecology practice in 2010, around the same time her bleeding started getting worse. The lack of access to consistent gynecology care would have major consequences on her health.

In 2012, two years after her gynecologist left, Ms. Barbara found another one to see. It didn't go well. "Sometimes, you know, you find a doctor, you think it's gonna be okay. But . . . you can tell them what's going on . . . and . . ." she trails off. "They don't really go into the questioning. It's just 'you'll be all right,' you know." She told the doctor that she was still having periods and that they were getting heavier. She asked if that was normal. I wish I could have been a fly on the wall in this conversation to understand what went wrong. Though it is uncomfortable to be so forward with someone I respect, I press Ms. Barbara for details. Here's what she remembers: The doctor was a White woman from California. She said to Ms. Barbara, "Well, maybe we should just go in your uterus and take part of it." "She wanted to do a D&C?" I ask. No, Ms. Barbara is sure she didn't use that phrase. "A biopsy?" No, Ms. Barbara is sure she didn't use that word either, because it would have scared her, she tells me. (I'm almost certain the doctor was referring to an endometrial biopsy with the words *piece of your uterus,* but that doesn't matter, because Ms. Barbara is the one who needed to have understood, and she didn't.) Ms. Barbara was actually open to the idea of this next step to "take a part of her uterus," but was thinking that her Pap tests had always been normal and she'd just had another one that day with this new doctor. She'd wait to see about the results of the Pap first and then perhaps set up this next step for her next annual exam. She didn't know the Pap smear is not made to evaluate the causes of abnormal bleeding. So, when her Pap results came back normal, she was reassured. When she called the next year for her appointment, ready for the "piece of your uterus" test, she learned the doctor had left and gone back to California. Another ob-gyn had closed shop and left town.

While Ms. Barbara is talking, I am having a full-body reaction and working hard not to show it. Inside, I am quaking with frustration. Ms. Barbara is an employed, insured woman fully active and engaged with the healthcare system. She took her medicine, she followed up, and, amazingly, she actually disclosed her bleeding symptoms despite being met with minimal concern. Thus far, no one has said the words *endometrial cancer* to her. No one has pressed her on the critical nature of a biopsy. No one has even told her that this increasingly heavy bleeding, in her sixties, is not normal. She saw three different (non-gynecology) doctors on a regular basis that took great care of her other medical conditions and didn't ask about anything below the belt. She kept working, and she kept bleeding.

The research theory and framework that guides how I ask scientific questions is called the Public Health Critical Race praxis, developed by Dr. Chandra Ford and Dr. Collins Airhihenbuwa. It is an adaptation of critical race theory, which was first pioneered in legal studies and then education, before this application to public health. The praxis emphasizes that groups at the "margins," those who are doing the worst, should be at the center of research efforts. I believe this focus is one of this framework's most important offerings and is incredibly useful for scientific discovery. We don't just center the margins because it's the right thing to do, we center the margins because—medically—when you focus on the most vulnerable to the problem you want to address (e.g., death from endometrial cancer), you *will* also address each of the ways *anyone* can be vulnerable.* If the medical community had placed Black women at the center of its ef-

* Some readers will be most familiar with this idea from the Combahee River Collective statement: "If Black women were free, it would mean that everyone else would have to be free since our freedom would necessitate the destruction of all the systems of oppression." Amen.

forts five decades ago when the data made their needs clear, how well developed and targeted might endometrial cancer research, public health campaigns, workforce development, and prevention efforts be across the board? I don't know. Instead, I am acutely aware of the abysmal state we're in.

Black women have worse cases of endometrial cancer, and that reality is intertwined with others outlined in this book. We suffer more with endometrial cancer for the same reason Black women have worse fibroids that start earlier, grow bigger, and last longer. The same reason Black women have worse periods with heavier bleeding dysfunction and more profound anemia. Name a womb condition and the story is the same. Research that acknowledges these stark truths will be the only research that results in tangible, actual healing for the Black womb, and this is why it is the kind of work I do.

We have long known Black women are more likely to get these fast-growing, malignant tumors, so you might assume the medical community is on high alert to screen older Black women, identifying risk factors and detecting disease even before there are symptoms. You might assume there's an elaborate and detailed screening process in place to catch endometrial cancer in Black women as early as possible, evaluate them promptly, and maximize the chance of survival. Sadly, you would be wrong.

Black women are consistently diagnosed at more advanced stages of endometrial cancer than White women. This is true across different hospital systems and geographic regions and regardless of insurance type. One of my earlier research studies in this area was evaluating more than 4,500 women with Medicare insurance who go to the doctor. Every woman was insured and had healthcare access. Black women were still twice as likely to be diagnosed with stage IV endometrial cancer. This was one of the big signals to me that there was a problem with how we diagnose endometrial cancer altogether.

We mostly diagnose cancers through biopsy. That's true whether the cancer is in your colon, your neck, or your uterus. We need to get a sample of the tissue and look at it under a microscope. Often, we also need to send it for genetic analysis. That's how we know if a blip on an ultrasound or shadowing on a CT scan is something benign or cancer. A cancer in your womb is no different.

But in the 1990s, something significant happened in my field of gynecology. We moved away from using a biopsy as the initial approach to diagnosis, delaying that step until other potential problems are ruled out. We can't yet screen for endometrial cancer (detect it before there are any symptoms), so we wait until the patient starts reporting symptoms. At that time, studies (many of which exclusively included White women) showed that 90 percent of endometrial cancer had the same symptom: postmenopausal bleeding, or bleeding after the menopause transition is complete. But postmenopausal bleeding can also be caused by benign polyps, fibroids that poke into the uterine cavity, or endometrial thinning from age or menopause. How could doctors avoid an invasive and often painful biopsy for people who were bleeding abnormally, but not because of cancer? The medical community put one more step in place: an ultrasound to review how thick the patient's endometrium is.* If a transvaginal ultrasound revealed that a patient's endometrial thickness was less than 4 mm, then there was pretty much no chance of endometrial cancer. The American College of Obstetricians and Gynecologists (ACOG) and many other clinical organizations endorsed this research and adopted this ultrasound-based triage process. There was no reason for biopsy unless repeated episodes of bleeding occurred.

The change was well intentioned and meant to spare cancer-free women from an uncomfortable procedure. This is a fine strategy if the patient in question is at low risk for aggressive endometrial cancer. It's also a fine strategy if the endometrial thickness test is highly accurate. Both are true of White women. Also, most of the studies that demonstrated the efficacy of ultrasound testing were done on them.

* See chapter 3, "The Basics," for a review of the endometrium—the innermost wall of the uterus.

But neither circumstance is true for Black women, who are at high risk for aggressive endometrial cancer. A missed diagnosis is a major problem when you have a fast-growing disease. Through my research studies, we learned that this ultrasound test was not nearly as accurate in Black women. In fact, this test missed almost 10 percent of Black women with endometrial cancer. A test designed to minimize biopsies was geared toward the experiences of White women and has led to missed diagnoses in Black women and subsequent lethal consequences. Prioritizing White comfort at the expense of Black lives is not new in our society. Even for me, it's easy to get lost in the numbers and the data of this inequity, but stories like Ms. Barbara's remind me of what is at stake.

As she continues with her story, Ms. Barbara has my full attention. It is now 2014, and she continues to bleed. She's sixty-four years old. It's been two years since her last gynecology visit, four years since she noticed her bleeding getting heavier, and she's starting to get annoyed. She was beginning to have unexpected "gushes" at work, with no indication of when they would happen. She had a positive and long-standing relationship with the doctor she saw for her thyroid, an endocrinologist named Dr. Murray. He was the person who, many years earlier, had taken her breathing problems seriously and got her in to see the cardiologist who quickly diagnosed and treated her heart failure. Of all the providers she saw, she was most comfortable with Dr. Murray, an older White man. So, during a visit that year, she told him that she was getting "tired of all the bleeding and clots and surprises at work." And God bless this man, because he responded with appropriate alarm. He wondered immediately if she needed a hysterectomy. Perhaps we can all now understand why this suggestion sounded wild to Ms. Barbara. "A hysterectomy?! I told him no because I always get my Paps and they are always fine." Dr. Murray, who I appreciate more and more as I listen, didn't let it go. He told her that she at least needed a D&C because, at her age, she shouldn't be bleeding anymore. She listened to him because she trusted him. He had earned that trust by showing her care and believing her time and again over the years. She once again set out to find a new gynecologist, one she could have for the long term. This time, she asked her friend for a recommendation. When she called that provider's office, they were not taking new patients.

Ms. Barbara was trying to follow through on Dr. Murray's advice, but her efforts got delayed. She had no idea that she was having the number one symptom of endometrial cancer, though. She also had a lot of other things going on. She was working full-time, was running her Simply Soulful Café on the side, and had become the primary caregiver for her treasured, ailing mother. Ms. Barbara's mom, who at the time still lived independently in Spokane, Washington, had an accumulation of mini-strokes from hypertension that turned into dementia. After Ms. Barbara heard one too many times from family and neighbors that her mother wasn't making sense or had been out in the road undressed and confused, Ms. Barbara moved her mother into her house in Seattle. She had now become a full-time caregiver in addition to her other jobs, ensuring her mother took her medications in the morning, arranging for home health visits during the day, and getting her plugged into the healthcare system in Seattle. Yes, Ms. Barbara cared about her own bleeding and wanted to see it stop, but in her mind, it was about her period and not about *cancer*. It could wait.

In 2016, on top of the bleeding, Ms. Barbara started to have pelvic and left-sided abdominal pain. She went to see her primary care physician about it and told him, "I don't know why I am still having a period. It's really frustrating to keep bleeding like this." He didn't have immediate thoughts but decided she should see a visiting nurse practitioner who came to the office once a week for gynecology-related issues. Ms. Barbara received a basic pelvic exam and recalls having an ultrasound that "came out okay," but the nurse practitioner recommended a biopsy. This provider took the time to clarify that despite her clear Paps, Ms. Barbara's bleeding and symptoms indicated the need for a biopsy. The NP called her back quickly with the results. Her biopsy showed *serous carcinoma,* one of the most aggressive and lethal forms of endometrial cancer. She gave Ms. Barbara a referral to a new gynecologic oncologist who had just recently begun practicing out of the nearby university hospital: Dr. Kemi M. Doll.

Ms. Barbara's journey in and out of offices demonstrates how the current process to diagnose endometrial cancer disserves Black women and, increasingly, everyone else.* We physicians assume women have a clear sign they're in menopause. Twelve months with no menstrual bleeding means perimenopause is over and they've officially crossed the threshold out of their reproductive years. But women of color, including Black women, have menopausal symptoms for longer than White women and often report longer periods of irregular bleeding phases. Under these circumstances, how does one know if bleeding is postmenopausal or not? We assume women in their sixties and seventies with irregular bleeding will run to the doctor for help, but Black women have legitimate reasons to be leery of providers. We Black women have a long history of and ongoing experience with receiving not help but trauma from gynecologic and reproductive healthcare providers in this country. Why would a few drops of blood make you put your dignity and bodily safety back in harm's way for a condition you've never heard of? Then there's the assumption that when Black women do share their symptoms, they are met with prompt attention and evaluation. Besides the obvious statistics that show many more advanced cancers among us, my research has also demonstrated that physicians are generally ill informed about endometrial cancer symptoms, risk, and appropriate diagnostic steps.

I don't think the question is "Why are Black women diagnosed at more advanced stages of endometrial cancer?" or "Why has their cancer spread more when they finally get a diagnosis?" Instead, the question the medical and public health communities should be asking is "When are we going to prioritize the early detection of endometrial

* ACOG has reaffirmed its position on transvaginal ultrasound as an initial test for endometrial cancer in 2018 and again in 2023, despite mounting evidence that it underserves Black women. At the time of this writing, I've been told that this position is currently under review.

cancer in Black women and start saving lives?" The answer must be "Now."

One way we categorize how quickly a cancer is expected to attack and spread throughout a patient's body is by looking at its cells under a microscope.* In very broad terms, there are two categories of endometrial cancer—type 1 and type 2. In type 1, the cancer tissue is similar to the original endometrial womb tissue in its healthy state. Type 1 is slow growing and mostly comes from having too much estrogen in your body. This hormonal overload is either generated internally (i.e., from fat cells or an estrogen-producing ovarian or adrenal tumor, common in younger folks) or externally (i.e., from taking too much estrogen in hormone replacement therapy without any balancing progesterone, common in older folks). The endometrial tissue is sensitive to estrogen, and if you overload it, it can transform into type 1 endometrial cancer.

In White women, endometrial cancer is usually Type 1.

Type 2 endometrial cancer is quite different. For one, it is *not* primarily fueled by hormones. Under a microscope, type 2 endometrial cancer does *not* look like regular endometrial tissue. It has extremely aggressive molecular mutations—namely, a mutation of the tumor suppressor gene *TP53*.† Endometrial cancers that fall in this type 2 category are called *serous, carcinosarcoma,* and *clear cell*. From the time we started naming and measuring them, they have been found in greater numbers in Black women. They don't care what your body size is. They don't care how many babies you've had or whether

* This is called *histology,* and the medical specialists who undertake the investigation are called *pathologists*. Cancers are grouped into histology types, and those categories tell us which cancers need more treatment (e.g., chemotherapy or radiation) than others.

† The normal function of *TP53* is to keep cells' frequent genetic errors from transforming into cancer. People who have *TP53* mutations get many cancers throughout their lives and often die quite young because their *TP53* throughout their bodies does not work properly. When a certain kind of tissue gets a *TP53* mutation, it becomes high risk for cancer. Most type 2 endometrial cancers have serious *TP53* mutations.

you've given birth at all. They don't care what kind of sex you've had or when. They are aggressive cancers that grow in the womb. Among all populations in the United States, Black women are uniquely at risk, and twice as likely to get these types as anyone else.* Understanding why this is the case, as of 2025, is a major area of research. We have signals from other diseases that *TP53* mutations are acquired throughout life, and the strongest driver is age. The older you are, the more opportunity there has been for the *TP53* gene to make a natural mistake and become mutated. (This is why endometrial cancer strikes later in life, in the menopausal years.) What if there are other factors, however, that increase the likelihood of those natural mistakes, making them occur sooner? In a small research study I co-conceived with Dr. Rosana Risques, Dr. Eric Rios-Doria, and Dr. Elizabeth Swisher, we found that *TP53* mutations in normal endometrial tissue clearly increase with age in both Black and White women. Our sample was too small to know if these mutations happen earlier in Black women, though there were some early markers that Black women may accumulate more *TP53* "hot spot" mutations in the years preceding endometrial cancer. Part of my current thinking on this is that given that Black women are exposed to more environmental pollutants, more childhood adversity, more chronic stress, and, specifically, more gynecologic stress over their lifetimes—there is something in this mix that increases our vulnerability to *TP53* mutations and leads to patterns we see in endometrial cancer. This aligns with research on other women of color that demonstrates that endometrial cancer is, on average, diagnosed at earlier ages among Native American and Latina women as well. This is where I want to see much more research.

---

* Recently, there have been advances to characterize endometrial cancer beyond what we can see under the microscope. We can use the DNA of the tumors themselves to know which endometrial cancers are aggressive or not. When we use these molecular categories—there are four of them—the most aggressive is called *Copy Number High*. Its distinguishing feature? *TP53* mutations. The population with the most Copy Number High class of endometrial cancer? Black women. The pattern is always the same.

When I met Ms. Barbara, I was fresh out of my fellowship, had passed my board exam with all these memorized types of endometrial cancer swirling in my head, and was in my first year of independent practice. She was on my schedule as a "NEW PATIENT—UTERINE CANCER." We were scheduled for an hour-long visit, and I knew we needed to cover a lot of ground. I had her medical records that showed her positive biopsy for cancer. I knew from her cancer type she would need chemotherapy and radiation after surgery. And I knew she was Black. This visit would set the tone of her entire cancer journey. I knew that I would give her my absolute best. She represented the reason I had spent sixteen years of my life getting to this point. I walked in, smiled, and introduced myself. I asked Ms. Barbara what she remembers of our meeting.

"Oh my goodness, I had not known you were Black! I was so, so relieved," she tells me now. "I knew I was in trouble, and I just didn't know how I was going to take care of this on top of everything else. But once you walked in, I said to myself, 'I'm going to do whatever she tells me to do.' "

I smile as she shares her recollections. I remember a regal, older Black woman who was so composed and gave me her absolute attention. I remember her saying that her cancer was *her fault* and me feeling so angry in response that I actually interrupted her and declared that it absolutely was *not*. I remember talking gently about the aggressiveness of her cancer type and how we really needed to get to surgery as soon as possible. I had to swallow my frustration when she agreed but told me we had to cancel the date I had already reserved for her because she had to find someone to take care of her ailing mother. We pushed her surgery back another month.

Ms. Barbara had surgery in the spring of 2017. I admit I don't remember her actual surgery because it went smoothly. I performed a minimally invasive (robotic) cancer surgery for her, the gold standard procedure for her diagnosis. As with most surgeons, what sticks in my mind are the harrowing cases, not the uneventful ones that go as planned. One of the reasons I chose to work at a major academic medical center was because of their excellent surgical care team and top-of-the-line facilities. You can be an excellent surgeon, but if you have a terrible team, the patient is in danger. By the time I took Ms. Barbara to the operating room, I had a great relationship with my team, which was made up of surgical nurses, OR techs, and medical trainees. We removed her uterus, tubes, ovaries, and lymph nodes. We also sampled other tissue areas, which is standard as part of a comprehensive endometrial cancer surgery. I was disappointed but not surprised when her pathology results showed the cancer was in nearly every single specimen we removed. The surgery was just the beginning.

With her list of medical conditions and her age, I was worried about Ms. Barbara getting through surgery, then chemotherapy, then radiation. She ended up being surprised that going through treatment wasn't nearly as bad as she was warned about. She didn't get very sick with chemotherapy; she just felt tired. She loved the oncology treatment team, including our exceptional head nurse, Holly Tomashek, who would visit Ms. Barbara's restaurant during off-hours (and still does to this day). I'm glad her memory has smoothed out the rough edges of her treatment journey. I know I watched her chemotherapy doses like a hawk, attuned to the ways the medications might interact with her other conditions. After her third or fourth dose, she got short of breath and required a brief hospital stay, during which her heart medications were readjusted. I was terrified, but Ms. Barbara barely remembers that. She remembers being cared for and surviving.

Ms. Barbara's treatment success was the result of science. The science surrounding cancer treatments can stay stagnant for decades, then make breathtaking leaps forward in a few years. Endometrial cancer treatment is no exception. In 2023, at the Society of Gynecologic Oncology's Annual Meeting on Women's Cancer, there were two jaw-dropping presentations reporting on two different new medications that improved overall survival rates for endometrial cancer patients. Women with advanced cancer, previously expected to survive only a few months, were alive and thriving years later. There were standing ovations and even some tears. It had been two decades since new medications successfully targeted endometrial cancer. Finally, we were making headway. Discussion of this cancer used to be relegated to a single session amid a five-day scientific conference. Today, endometrial cancer dominates the prime presentation slots, with a growing number of studies and progress in treatment each year. I will not do a deep dive into all the potential endometrial cancer treatments, as it's quite likely that by the time you read these words, some existing protocols will already be out of date. My unabashed hope is to restore Black women to a place of uterine balance, and that means when Black women are diagnosed with endometrial cancer, I want us to have cutting-edge treatment and keep going with our important, valuable lives.

I don't want us to be scared of cancer treatment. The traditional chemotherapy agents are meant to destroy fast-growing cells and often have natural origins. Paclitaxel comes from the Pacific yew tree, native to the Pacific Northwest in North America, and is also found in Europe and Japan. It has been a compound used in traditional healing practices of Native American, First Nation, and Japanese peoples and likely more communities that have gone undocumented in history. It is now synthesized in a way that preserves the antitumor effect while minimizing the ecological harm of harvesting from trees. Carboplatin destroys mutated DNA common in cancer cells. It is a form of the naturally occurring metal platinum, which you may remember from the periodic table of elements in eighth-grade science class. Platinum has existed on this planet millions of years longer than humanity has, and we have discovered how to modify this gift from Mother Earth to target cancer cells in the body. When we live in a world of us versus them ("natural" versus "synthetic" or "pharmaceutical," "herbs" versus "drugs," etc.), we lose nuance and, frankly, facts. These two compounds are the backbone of endometrial cancer treatment, and I used them countless times to cure my patients.

Now we also have newer targeted treatments that take different routes. Immunotherapy adds signals to cancer cells so our immune system can more easily find them. VEGF inhibitors cut off the blood supply to cancer cells so they starve and die. Gene therapy and tumor vaccines identify the molecular fingerprints of cancer cells and shut down the mutations that keep them alive. The world of cancer treatment is vast and ever changing. It is a world that Black women need not fear. Women with advanced-stage cancers who were all but certain to die within a year are living so long that they are shutting down the trials designed to measure length of survival. This is not everyone's story, but it is a real beginning. And it is enough to keep us all pushing to ensure that Black women know not just what endometrial cancer is and how to identify its symptoms but the wealth of treatment options available. I am so grateful Ms. Barbara trusted me. Because she trusted me and completed her treatment, she lived.

~

As we sit in my living room, I ask Ms. Barbara to share any other insights from her cancer experience. "I still feel like I neglected myself. I didn't take time to just really study up on what was going on. I put it to the side to just keep going, you know?" she tells me. I do know. And I know that Ms. Barbara, like any other Black woman, shouldn't have to bear this burden; I know that a Black woman actively managing her conditions, dutifully going to all her doctors' appointments, running a thriving business, and caring for her family should not have had to add "uterine bleeding investigator" to her job list. She should not have had suspicious bleeding for four years and gone without a diagnosis until she had the kind of pain and increased bleeding that indicated her cancer was spreading. That was my profession's job. That was *our* job. And we failed her.

Today, Ms. Barbara is a kindhearted woman who talks about her grandchildren and her "grandpuppies" with equal fondness. I could sit and talk with her all day. I ask her if there's anything else she wants to tell me. "I'm just so grateful to be alive, every day I wake up. I just want to live the dream, make somebody laugh, and make somebody's day." I thank God I crossed paths with Ms. Barbara. She continues to be a blessing to her family, her community, and, hopefully, everyone reading these words.

~

Not everyone makes it.

Often, endometrial cancer strikes down Black women in their fifties, sixties, and seventies, just as they're reaching the full expression of their immense wisdom. Often, they have accumulated power from lifetimes spent strategizing how to live in a country that hates them. Their gifts are finally in full bloom. Maya Angelou wrote "Still I Rise" and "Phenomenal Woman" at age fifty. Supreme Court Justice Ketanji Brown Jackson was nominated to our highest court in the land at fifty-one. Oprah Winfrey launched her own network, OWN, four weeks before her fifty-seventh birthday. Vice President Kamala Harris was the presidential nominee at age sixty. Toni Morrison won the Nobel Prize for literature at sixty-two. Losing Black women in this iridescent phase of glory is a complete and utter tragedy. Far too often, our matriarchs are stolen from us while in their prime.

Gwen Ifill was anchor of *PBS NewsHour* and a prescient political thinker who predicted Kamala Harris's rise to success. The legendary Black political journalist died in November 2016 of endometrial cancer, just a year after diagnosis. There are many more Black women and their family members I could list as being touched by this illness, but their diagnoses are private and I respect their families' choices to simply offer "cancer" as the cause of death. But I can't help but wonder if the below-the-belt location of endometrial cancer makes this vagueness more appealing. Even in death, the silencing and shame continue. Strictly by looking at national statistics, I know there must be many prominent Black women who have had endometrial cancer or are going through treatment for it. I hope this book, and this chapter especially, serve as a call to come forward and help bring this common and dangerous disease into the light.

Dr. Tiffany Nicole Jones is a young emerging endometrial cancer scientist who I respectfully refer to as our "Shuri of Wakanda," as she is whip-smart and just as charming. She is untangling the mystery of stress, race, and endometrial cancer through molecular studies and epigenetics *while still in medical training* to become a gynecologic oncologist. Her life partner is Shakiya Canty, a divinity school graduate and community organizer. Shakiya's grandmother Ellen died of endometrial cancer in 2018. I spoke with Shakiya and her mother, Tikiya, at length about their matriarch Ms. Ellen and was thrilled to sit down with a mother-daughter pair.

We meet on Zoom over the holidays in the fall of 2024, when Shakiya is back home in Philly and they can be together in person. They describe Ms. Ellen as a natural caregiver whom babies loved and whose hair-care skills made her a highly sought-after stylist in the family. "Everyone would be over at our house on Saturday waiting for her hot comb," Tikiya recalls with fondness and a smile. "She could really make hair grow." Ms. Ellen and her husband had suffered tragedy when they tried to start a family. They lost their first and only biological pregnancy to miscarriage when Ms. Ellen was nearly five months along. She never discussed it, but Tikiya knew it was a place of tender grief for her mother. A few years later, Ms. Ellen adopted Tikiya, who was the infant granddaughter of an auntlike figure in Ms. Ellen's life. Ms. Ellen was thrilled to take in and raise Tikiya. The adoption of a distant relation or young community member was common in West Philly at this time, when folks didn't have much but everyone cared for one another.

Ms. Ellen taught a growing Tikiya how to care for herself and her gynecologic health in the way Ms. Ellen knew best. Unfortunately, this knowledge was not born of science but of family traditions passed down from an earlier time. Tikiya was taught to shave her private areas, to regularly douche, and to even use suppositories all in service of vaginal health. These things are not needed and are more likely to cause infections and chronic irritation than give any benefit.*

The details Tikiya shares are interesting to me, because in most of the stories I've collected, it's rare a mother offers this level of gynecology advice. Typically, there's silence about gynecologic health, other than teaching how to manage the blood. In this case, Ms. Ellen was quite involved and active in teaching her daughter to

* If you are worried about odor, use an external perfume. The vagina (inner canal beyond the labial folds) is a self-cleaning oven. It doesn't need anything up there. If you have recurrent yeast infections, there is a well-developed, well-researched medical protocol to help you. Go see a board-certified gynecologist and make sure you detail your full history to get put on the right treatment pathway. The medication, dose, and frequency differ depending on your personal history.

prioritize her gynecologic health. The information was just misguided.

Because of stories like these and the explosion of social media content from Black women seeking to help others navigate womb health, I reject the traditional medical narrative that Black people disregard our health. What is true is that despite a natural desire to be well and a strong tradition of passing down the tools for survival from mother to daughter and beyond, we don't always have the right information. We aren't targeted well by public health campaigns. We are left out of important clinical trials. When we share the intimate details of our health in doctors' offices, we are often met with disregard, apathy, or outright suspicion. I don't know the origin of every practice Ms. Ellen taught her daughter in the 1980s, but I know they were born in a period where Black women had to come up with many of their own solutions for their problems.

Tikiya tells me that Ms. Ellen went through menopause around age fifty. Around age sixty-six, Ms. Ellen told her daughter she was bleeding again. Tikiya doesn't know exactly when it started, but Ms. Ellen told her then "this wasn't the first time." Tikiya was worried and accompanied her mother to the doctor. During Ms. Ellen's biopsy a few visits later, Tikiya held her hand while tears rolled down her mother's face. The procedure was performed by a cold, unfeeling provider. "He seemed so mechanical. . . . He didn't even say 'We're almost done' or 'Hang in there' or anything like that," she tells me. "He was just getting the tools, doing what he needed to do, in silence. I felt so bad that I couldn't help her, just hold her hand."

Tikiya's recollections are important, but I have trepidation over including this part of Ms. Ellen's story. I worry it will scare anyone reading this and you might forgo an endometrial biopsy if you're referred for one. That's understandable. I don't know anyone excited about potential uterine pain. But Black women avoiding endometrial biopsies directly leads to more delayed diagnoses, more advanced cancer by the time it's found, and more dead Black matriarchs. This is the opposite of what I want and what we need. Endometrial biopsy can be very painful for some and feel like "a pinch" for others. Gynecologists can do things to help. They can use a paracervical block, in which a numbing agent is injected directly into the cervix first superficially, then, once that takes effect, deeper to get more numbness throughout. This can make a huge difference because a lot of the pain a patient experiences comes from the instrument we use to hold the cervix in place and from the cervical dilation. The actual biopsy pipette creates a small vacuum effect in the uterus and samples cells from the top to the bottom of the endometrial cavity.*

Dr. Linda Bradley, a preeminent Black gynecologist at the Cleveland Clinic, argues that all endometrial biopsies should be done with a camera, allowing the technician to visualize the uterus in real time. (This is called *hysteroscopy,* and Dr. Bradley is a pioneer in this technique.) I agree. We can get the best samples when we can see the endometrium, like a hysteroscopy allows. But most gynecologists' offices are not equipped to do hysteroscopy, as it usually requires sedation. It can also require general anesthesia and, if so, must be done in an operating room. In addition, hysteroscopy is much more expensive than an endometrial biopsy. Depending on insurance provider and quality, the cost could be prohibitive for many people.

I wish to live long enough to see this kind of gynecologic care provided with no financial barrier. I wish to see the many potentially painless new endometrial cancer diagnostic tests be fully developed and replace the biopsy. But for now, here's my honest take: a biopsy can be painful. Biopsy is also not perfect—you need a skilled provider to do one and a knowledgeable physician to interpret the results. If not enough tissue is taken to understand what is going on, some folks will need a D&C and further testing. However, biopsy is also quick, done in a doctor's office, and, very critically, can (and should) be done with extreme kindness and support. Most importantly, it is worth it to know whether you have a cancer that is still curable when diagnosed early. Instead of enduring severe symptoms for weeks, months, or years, I'd rather we endure much less pain for a much shorter time when undergoing the tests and procedures that provide

* There is a common misconception that the biopsy only takes tissue from one place. When done properly, it actually siphons off cells from the fundus (top of uterus) down to the cervix. Doing two or three passes is important for getting a solid sample, and a pass is relatively quick, about three seconds.

the knowledge we can use to save our own lives. And I know we know how to do that.

Ms. Ellen would end up being diagnosed with stage IIIC endometrial cancer, serous (high-risk) type. But unlike my patient Ms. Barbara, who had nearly the same diagnosis and stage, Ms. Ellen didn't make it. After a successful initial treatment in 2015, her cancer came back in 2018, and she passed that April, a month before her seventieth birthday. Tikiya was one of her primary caretakers. To this day, Tikiya keeps in her medicine cabinet one dose of the daily heparin shots she had to give her mother, "for nostalgic purposes."

What did we lose when Ms. Ellen died? "A matriarch," Tikiya says. "She was hooked on phonics before Hooked on Phonics was a thing. She taught all the neighborhood kids how to read. She was always caring for everyone's children. Just always there for people, with a house full of kids."

Shakiya, Ms. Ellen's granddaughter, has been so quiet throughout this conversation that we set up a time to meet again, just the two of us. During that session, she agrees with her mother that we lost an incredible nurturer and a leader when Ms. Ellen died. As a community organizer, Shakiya knows how critical the kind of care her grandmother provided really is. "Think about a single mom or struggling family," she says. For them, Ms. Ellen's presence in the community meant "the difference between them being able to have her as a backup for the kids versus not. All that knowledge she had to pass down is just gone."

I ask Shakiya about her own womb-health journey, and she admits it's still in progress. As a queer Black woman, a Christian, and a divinity school grad pastor turned community organizer, she's been unpacking her connection to her womb for several years. Her only goal growing up in the church was not to get pregnant. "I remember I was afraid to turn eighteen, because that's when a lot of my family members got pregnant. I didn't know that wasn't something to be ashamed of, because there was so much focus on it being sinful. My grandma used to say, 'While climbing the ladder of success, don't let the boys look up your dress.'" Her words remind me of how much we emphasize contraceptive protection and not holistic gynecologic health. The most enduring message Shakiya carries leaves out the very knowledge needed to prevent another endometrial cancer death in the family. She admits our conversation with her mother, Tikiya, about her grandmother Ms. Ellen was a revelation to her. "I'm still processing," she concludes.

To me, this is the power of womb stories and why I suggest in part 3 of this book the deliberate telling and sharing of these intimate journeys with our true friends. There is something profound about how following the story of your womb connects you to so many important moments of your life and reveals your way of connecting to your own body. The womb is powerful.

Medical advances are not the only area where progress is being made in endometrial cancer. There's been progress on the public health front in recent years, and I'm proud that Black women have been at the forefront. In 2016, I met and immediately bonded with a towering figure in the Black breast cancer advocacy space, Ms. Bridgette Hempstead. Bridgette, a survivor of metastatic breast cancer herself, had founded Cierra Sisters, an advocacy and support group for Black women with breast cancer in the Seattle and Puget Sound region. She was the ultimate cheerleader, community connector, and mentor to me, an enthusiastic but naive new physician and researcher. With her encouragement, I asked one of my first patients, Marjorie (Margie) Willis, to partner with me to start something that didn't exist for endometrial cancer—a support and advocacy organization for Black women. Margie's story is another extraordinary one. She is a former fitness instructor, healthy food guru, and vivacious grandmother who was diagnosed with endometrial cancer at fifty-eight. She is four foot, ten inches, with a slim build and better cardiovascular fitness than mine. (She, along with many others like her, is the reason I will not lead with obesity in any message about endometrial cancer for Black women. Is it a factor? Sure. Is it the only or the most important factor for Black folks? *No.*) Together with two of my amazing research staff members, Liz Sage and Julianna Alson, supporting us, Ms. Bridgette, Margie, and I co-founded ECANA (Endometrial Cancer Action Network for African Americans). Our first step was to recruit brave Black endometrial cancer survivors who could encourage a new kind of strength in their peers, one rooted in community and a reclamation of their own stories of navigating the illness.

The day-to-day work of launching ECANA involved grant writing, recruiting the support of my professional organization of gynecologic oncologists, and casting a wide net for community outreach. In those early years, we got pushback because of our focus on Black women. On a critical call to gain the support of the Society of Gynecologic Oncology, we heard, "Why just Black women? Why don't you help everyone?" We all knew the answer: because we can and should focus on Black women. Black women specifically had been left behind and left to die. We stood our ground and pushed ahead, and many of my colleagues expressed support at critical junctures, writing letters of support and joining our advisory board. These important endorsements led to our successful grant funding and allowed us to launch. In doing this, I believe we were actively shifting our community's strength from denial and silent endurance to renewal and reclamation. We launched a website and quickly recruited more Black women endometrial cancer survivors to be peer educators and break the silence on bleeding and endometrial cancer risks for older women. These ECANA ambassadors focused on small, intimate settings where women could open up and be real. They got to work redefining gynecologic health norms among their friends and families. Another major priority of ECANA was training our ambassadors to be research consultants and partner with science teams to ensure their studies were inclusive and respectful of Black women. As a lone researcher, I could not answer all the questions remaining about how to save Black women with endometrial cancer, and I was tired of seeing research on us, without us. These ECANA community research consultants' work filled this gap. ECANA's community education, peer support, and research partnership continues today with the addition of national advocacy campaigns and lobbying efforts.

After running ECANA for five years, in 2022, I stepped down to meet the final personal goal I had for the organization, which was to ensure it was led by the survivors themselves. The torch was passed to Adrienne Moore,* an early ECANA member and absolute powerhouse of an advocate, writer, and leader. I am so proud of ECANA as the work continues.

* Adrienne is yet another Black woman who doesn't fit expectations about who gets endometrial cancer. Diagnosed in her forties, she was working as a respiratory therapist, not obese, and very health conscious. She was diagnosed with stage III endometrial cancer after several trips to the emergency room and an ultrasound that was deemed "fine." Because Adrienne went through chemotherapy and radiation, she is still here. Because we continue to perpetuate a narrow view of what causes endometrial cancer, stories like hers of delayed and surprise diagnoses continue.

Part III

HOW WE HEAL

Changing the Script

CHAPTER 8

STRENGTH TO HEAL THE BLACK WOMB

HEALING OURSELVES

Let's heal. Now.

Any purported effort to take Black women's health seriously is incomplete without a focus on gynecologic health. To commit to healing Black wombs, we must commit to breaking generational patterns of suppression and silence.

For some of us, taking our womb health seriously is the first step to reconnecting to our bodies and our overall health. Too many Black women stop feeling and responding to our bodies' signals because we are desperately busy and overburdened by the pull of work and family. We are not intentionally choosing to neglect ourselves. We meet the needs of bosses, children, spouses, aging parents, family, and community. And once everyone else's demands are met, there just isn't time left over to think about or care for ourselves. "Keep it movin'" and "I don't have time for this" become unspoken mantras. If you find yourself in this group, I welcome you to use your pursuit of gynecologic health as the first step to reintegrating your physical well-being with the rest of your life. You may be twentysomething and feeling invincible or fortysomething and feeling over it all, but in either case, I promise your body has information for you. Our wombs hold volumes.

There's another group of us—those who have already divested from self-neglect and taken action to prioritize their self-care and rest. If you're reading this book, you may be more likely to fall into this category. Maybe you've even successfully broken the superwoman habit of self-denial and prioritizing a show of strength at your own expense. Still, you may have left the womb behind. It's understandable given the messages we receive from mothers, cousins, friends, and the healthcare system. We're told our suffering is normal. The severity of our symptoms and the disruption they cause are dismissed. It's easy to feel that gynecology providers see us only through the lens of pregnancy or infection. Many times, they don't really see us at all. If what I'm describing sounds familiar, welcome. Let's put the last puzzle piece—your gynecologic health—into that formidable self-care routine you've developed and break this pattern for ourselves and our children.

Last but not least are those who have come to this book with a preexisting practice of integrating womb health into your well-being. You've known nothing in this country was built for you, including gynecology, so you've turned to older wisdom practices and trial and error. You've taken diagnosis and treatment into your own hands. It is my hope that you'll find meaning in these pages as well. Womb warriors, I want to ensure you can take advantage of gynecology as you so desire. I want your decisions to be informed by evidence and understanding and not myth and fear. We are sovereign over our bodies and deserve access to all manners of healing.

WOMB SISTERS

Black sisterhood is special. I know because for most of my childhood and adolescence, I didn't have it. A major reason I pledged Delta Sigma Theta Sorority, Inc., in college was to experience this powerful and unique sisterhood. I gained fourteen line sisters* and began learning about Black female friendship. Yet I was also still learning so much about myself and navigating the turmoil of my home instability and academic failures. I held many impenetrable boundaries, and forming intimate friendships was a very slow process for me. Now, many years later, I still have those relationships, and I am grateful every day for their richness, warmth, and strength. I am in the company of women I respect and admire, and I trust that they feel the same about me. My inner child, who was so sure she had to change, radically, to ever be fully loved, is being healed through these friendships. So, I am coming from a place of reverence for Black sisterhood when I say: *We can do even better.*

I want us to move from good girlfriends and best friends or even sisters to Womb Sisters. How do we get there? The first step is sharing our womb stories. Speaking as a Black woman gynecologic oncologist, uterine cancer scientist, and careful interviewer for the powerful stories in this book—I can tell you that sharing your womb story is transformative. Taking action to intentionally counter the silence we have been taught to hold about our wombs is revolutionary. And when we do this within our Black sisterhoods, it creates even deeper and more indelible bonds. Our womb experiences are often connected to important moments in our lives, important values we've inherited, and the current way we think of our bodies. When we share womb stories, we share ourselves at a whole new level of vulnerability. We also create another layer of relational accountability, opening the door for a friend to ask with genuine interest, *How is your womb, Sis?* Our love and care for one another reminds us that our wombs matter, that suffering in isolation doesn't need to continue just because that's what we're used to.

I heard this firsthand from my friend Jereshia Hawk. Jereshia is a one-of-a-kind dynamic and magnetic individual. She is the true ver-

* #8, Nucleus; F15: The Legacy Confirmed, Spring 2002; The LEGENDARY Lambda Omega Chapter. #DukeDelta. Extra for life.

sion of someone who created something—a big, beautiful, dynamic life—from humble beginnings and plenty of intergenerational pain. Jereshia's story is hers to tell (and I hope she does; it could be a movie). Just as I learn from her, she learns from me. She's been present when I've offered Womb Wisdom in both professional and more informal settings. She's one of the many women who have been on the receiving end of one of my spontaneous markers-on-the-whiteboard motivational womb anatomy presentations.* Recently, Jereshia left me a voice note that moved me. She said my words have had an impact, and now she's taking a different approach to seeking womb care. She's started asking her close friends about *their* womb health. When she left me this message, she reflected on how powerfully this element had influenced one friendship in particular. "I have known this friend literally since we were kids, and she is my girl. But this topic has opened up a whole new level of depth to our relationship." She saw her friend take agency over her womb health and stop unhealthy habits that had been long-standing issues. This did not surprise me, because I have seen the power of the womb to knit relationships together. I've seen it in my own life with my Womb Sisters. I've seen it in the strength of my relationship with my gynecologist, who I don't have to see frequently to feel how much safety and security is in our relationship. And I've seen it with ECANA, the first national advocacy organization for Black women with endometrial cancer, which has built the strongest sisterhood I have seen in advocacy spaces.

The work to heal our wombs need not and should not be done alone. There are lessons on the journey that we must learn as individuals, but even those can be brought back, shared, and healed with our Womb Sisters. Now, every acquaintance is not a friend and every friend is not a sister, so every sister is—not—a Womb Sister. Use your discretion and your inner knowing about who in your circle is ready for a deeper relationship.

Your womb sisterhood should not feel like a clique where you and your besties are all on the same program, doing the same things. To me, this is a dishonor to our individual family legacies and the matri-

* Worthy—if I may say so myself—of a TED Talk.

lineal heritage we carry. The meaning making we are tasked to do is unique and individual. The only clique or club I want us all to belong to is the one where we prioritize womb health. The specifics of what treatments or otherwise that are right for you don't have to be the same for your Womb Sisters. Save the clique energy for fashion, music, and the group chat. Womb health is too serious for this.

You can use the steps below as guidance, the agenda—if you will—for those dedicated times you meet up for Womb Talk with your Womb Sisters. Or you can make a commitment to have Womb Talk become part of your routine conversation. It may be a combination of both. I suggest at least one meeting dedicated to the womb, however, as the emotional weight of this work is undeniable.

LEARNING OUR FAMILIES' WOMB STORIES

Early messages about our wombs inform how we deal with all our health issues going forward. I can't tell you how many times I've gone to ask a sixty-plus-year-old Black woman about her uterine symptoms, and she starts telling me about how her mother, grandmother, foster mother, or older friend from down the block taught her (or didn't) about what to do (or not do) when "something's wrong down there." I want to get these stories out, on the table, and on the record. We must sort out wisdom from maladaptation, and sort out familial insights from generational trauma. If you can sit down with your family who raised you, here are some prompts to get started. Regardless, these are great topics for you and your Womb Sisters too.

- When did you start bleeding, and who took care of you?
- When did you stop bleeding, and what was that transition like? Who helped you?
- If you had a hysterectomy, when did that happen? Why did it happen?
- What is your womb health like now?
- Here is what it is like for me . . .

Ultimately, this is ancestral work. This is what I've found in my own experience speaking with the women in my family line who came before me. Through questions like those above, I learned about my grandmother's all-too-short life—and how it ended. I also learned about the emotional neglect my mother experienced as a grieving child and her own womb traumas. These stories led me to understand just how much my own womb health tied me to their lives. It gave me the motivation to break the Womb Suffering cycle just as much as I intend to break the other unhealthy cycles in our family. Too often, our lives are the culmination of denied and delayed dreams of generations of Black women who came before us. I encourage you to learn about your family history as a way to better understand your relationship to your own womb and your entitlement to self-care.

LEARNING OUR EMOTIONAL LANDSCAPE

I am a firm and ardent believer in therapy, specifically therapy received under the care of licensed mental health professionals who are Black women or women of color, or who have specific training and experience with marginalized races and genders in the United States. The strength of Black women will have us waiting to reach out for help until we are near the breaking point or past it. I know this because this was my experience.

The first time I walked into a therapist's office was the same day I learned that I would fail out of Duke University, where I was pursuing my undergraduate degree. In that office, I finally stopped pretending I could hold together my rapidly dissolving foundations after months of trying to cover up. I remember how stifled my voice was that day. I could barely get out my sentences for crying, while I was also unable to break my shell of strength to truly speak of my pain. It's hard to get anything out of therapy when you can't let your guard down. I didn't go back for over ten years.

As you now know, I got back on track academically and professionally with my tried-and-true strategy: outwork whatever challenge lay ahead of me. But at age thirty, when my husband and I confronted infertility, I met a challenge that couldn't simply be overcome with hard work and ambition. As those who have experienced this struggle know, infertility dissolves our illusions of control. Countless apps, herbal tinctures, gynecologic tests, and medical treatments promise a solution, but the person trying to conceive has no control over whether or not they actually work. Meanwhile, if you dare to share your struggle, you are often met with the callous and ignorant "It's just stress. Try not to think about it so much."*

For me, infertility was absolutely devastating. Of course, my professional life showed no evidence of the pressure I was under. I wrote and successfully won my first research grant. I successfully negotiated a novel arrangement between my clinical and research fellowships so I could complete the full requirements of both without shortchanging either. I showed up for my clinical duties every day, striving to be excellent for my patients. But inside, my sense of self was broken again, and I dragged myself into a therapist's chair.

I would stop and start therapy a few times as I finished my gynecologic oncology training and moved into motherhood. It wasn't until my second child, my daughter, was born that I came to understand that therapy was not just a way to manage my crises, it was for my routine everyday well-being. When I came to this realization, I was a surgeon, a scientist, and the mother of two children under four years old, married to an equally career-driven partner. Though I was not burned out in my career, I knew how easily I could head in that direction without a strong therapy support system. I was also determined to never view my children and my nurturing them as something at odds with my career ambition. I had heard an interview with Guy Johnson, Dr. Maya Angelou's son, during which he was asked what it was like to "grow up in her shadow." Angelou was so successful and had great ambition that took her around the world, and sometimes away from him. Johnson corrected the interviewer and shared the way he'd experienced his mother. "I did not have to grow

* Well-meaning people who say this, please listen to me when I tell you—it's not helpful. It's like telling someone who is appropriately upset and is experiencing something that you have not, to "calm down." If you think stress is contributing, ask yourself what you could do for your friend to lessen their stress, then do that.

up in her shadow. I was bathed in her light." His framing of the relationship gave me words for how I wanted my own children to experience me, with my ambition fully intact. It was then, when there were no fires to put out, that the real work in therapy began. I committed to tending to my mental and emotional health because I held such a desire to experience the fullness of life.

Unraveling memories and understanding the early ways I had adapted to survive as a child was transformative. I learned that I had the agency to move differently. My emotional vocabulary expanded from three modes (happy, angry, or tired) to a far more nuanced tapestry in which deeply felt joy could emerge as well. Therapeutic processes that have been invaluable in my life include Internal Family Systems work, somatic therapy, emotional freedom technique ("tapping"), and psychotherapy. Therapeutic guidance takes us from *living* our emotions to *understanding* our emotions. Understanding why we do things the way we do them helps us to reclaim our power and dignity. We can drop maladaptive defense mechanisms and leave unhelpful behaviors and relationships behind.

FEELING OUR BODIES AND OUR WOMBS

Our minds have a profound ability to disconnect from our bodies. Indeed, many of the stories you've read in these pages and the millions more represented by the statistics speak to Black women's breathtaking ability to disassociate from the womb and from ourselves. I believe this is a strength that has been bred into our lineage, allowing us to survive violence, pain, neglect, and dehumanizing experiences. Respectfully, it's time to stop seeing disassociation as a tool and to put it away. While there was a time when there was no help to be had for our wombs, times have now changed. We have a long way to go to an ideal gynecologic healthcare landscape, but there is a lot available to Black women right now. We can't access that care if we can't feel what is wrong. As you will see throughout this last section of the book and has been evident in many of the accounts you've read so far, most gynecologic treatment rests on a patient's insistence that something is wrong. There is no all-knowing test. It starts with us. And as Black women, we do know ourselves. We have had to recognize our own image and protect our self-knowledge against a racist and sexist world for generations. When it comes to your womb, there is no better expert than you.

But what if our lives are moving so fast and our minds are so busy that our bodies are an afterthought? Starting up any physical practice is a critical first step. We need times when we can escape the mind and remember that we are beings bound up in muscles, tissue, organs, and skin. It doesn't matter where we start, as long as we are forced into awareness of our bodies. We might be drawn to a daily walk, a fifteen-minute online yoga video, or a fancy new exercise bike. When we are talking about reconnection to the body, burning calories is irrelevant. Can you feel your limbs? Do you notice what aches when you've been sitting for too long? Can you feel that pressure in your pelvis? If so, is it worse than last year? If you're tired, does a nap help, or might that exhaustion be related to the bleeding that's lasted ten days?

If you are anything like me, used to moving quickly and letting your body catch up, this work of embodiment is not easy. I have coached hundreds of women of color* faculty in academic medicine, public health, and beyond who want to reach a new level of success. I stress with them the power of having the right frame of mind when we want to achieve a goal. Changing how we think and feel about a challenge can transform our experience and propel us to new heights. I know adopting a positive mindset isn't as easy as flipping a switch, so I often tell my clients, "If you can't figure out how to change your mind, commit to taking different action and let your mind catch up." I have similar advice for anyone seeking to reignite a connection to their physical body. You don't have to believe it's worth it. You can just get started and let the benefits catch up. Take that walk. Get on that bike. You may do it grudgingly now, but do it anyway and see how you feel in two weeks.

---

* I use the term *women of color* intentionally, as I coach Black, Latina, Asian, and Native American women in my company, not only Black women. When I am referring to Black women specifically, I say *Black*.

Perhaps you suffer from chronic pain or other comorbidities, and blocking out physical sensation is welcome. If so, this request to get into your body may seem ill advised. I do not have all the answers, and there may be latent ableism that I have not caught in these pages. I hope that by sharing my story, you will see a spark or seed of something you can apply to your own physical activity and movement journey.

I mention ableism because I have benefited from it. Not just because I am able-bodied in the general perspective of our society but also because I look fit. My body type is slim and muscular and it has been so my entire life, whether I was exercising twenty hours a week on my high school track-and-field team or existing off french fries, chocolate chip cookies, and full-calorie Coca-Cola for months during medical school and residency training. Regardless, people will say to me, "So, you run?" and "What kind of workouts do you do?" and, the worst, "You must be soooo disciplined."

I knew this was bias and privilege, but I didn't get a clock on how powerful it was until my late thirties, when I decided to commit myself to better physical health. Regardless of how I looked, I had high blood pressure that required two medications to control. I had very poor cardiovascular fitness, often huffing and puffing up the stairs. I'd had preeclampsia with both of my pregnancies and knew my lifetime risk of stroke or heart attack was uncomfortably high.

The first year of this commitment utterly failed, perhaps predictably. I set unrealistically high standards for myself, like not counting anything less than thirty minutes of sweating as a real workout. I set out to do things I hated, like running. Or I set up plans to do things I liked—hot yoga—but on a schedule that was too disruptive (midday on a weekday). I would stop and start, over and over, for years. In 2022, the year I turned forty, it finally turned around. Here's what I did:

I picked a time I could truly control, without any expectation of external demands. For me, that was 6:00–6:30 A.M.* I decided I

---

* Our kids get up at 6:00 to catch the bus around 7:00. My spouse does 6:00–6:30 A.M.; I do 6:30–7:00 A.M. Shout-out to all the parents and caregivers who climb a mountain of chaos before the workday begins.

would do something in that time frame that I didn't hate. Sweating was not a requirement. I started with some twenty-minute bike rides and short online yoga videos. I then added, slowly, some floor workouts for strength training. My goal was four days a week, to allow for ample misses. My goal changed from getting fit to simply being in my body. Success became putting on my workout clothes (which I laid out the night before and put right next to my bed), heading to my mat, and pushing Play. The habit stuck. Within those twenty-minute sessions, I began seeing improvement and feeling more and more energized. I could feel my body more, including subtle changes that helped me be more sensitive to my own body's cues. I could tell I was tired much sooner than I'd previously been able to, which helped me take breaks before I descended into total mental shutdown. My sleep improved and so did my discipline. This is what finally worked for me.

How is movement such a miracle drug? Sticking to this twenty-minute habit helped me to stick to other habits, like eating more fiber and having digital downtime each night. And of course, I came into greater awareness of my womb. I have a progesterone IUD, so I do not have a bleed each month. But I started to be able to feel when I had an ovulatory cycle anyway. I gained access to fantastic information for energy management and thinking about my menopausal transition.

Movement matters, and sadly, the hype is real. Making friends with routine and intentional movement has countless benefits. One of them is getting more in tune with the womb.

DON'T TRUST YOUR MEMORY— WRITE IT DOWN

When I was a medical student on the hospital wards, I learned something important about memory. My fellow trainees and I were usually the first in the room in the wee hours of the morning to touch base on each patient. I would ask people how their night was, did they pass gas, have they had any nausea, and so on. Prepared with their responses, I would go back to report to my supervisors before they then also entered the patient's room, usually an hour or more later. The patient's answers would often change when the doctors repeated the same questions I had asked. Yes, they did have some nausea and some pain on top of that, they might tell the attending physician. They hadn't lied to me. They just hadn't had a chance to really think about it. After being asked a second time, more details came to their minds. This is how memory works, and it is why I need you to start keeping a journal, log, or diary. It's not enough to depend on whatever random recollection of gynecologic symptoms come to mind during a scheduled appointment with your healthcare provider.

A journal will help you in three important ways. First, you will have an accurate record of your symptoms, which is critical to any medical evaluation and gives information about how and whether these symptoms require adaptation (or not) from you. Second, many Black women don't have access to a quality gynecology provider. Clinicians who don't specialize in women's health receive very little, if any, training on the topic. Also, Black women too often experience a lack of curiosity or empathy on the part of their providers, and systemic bias in the profession doesn't help. You may not have a doctor who asks a follow-up question or who circles back to ask you again and jog your memory. If all you are working with is a yes/no checklist from the waiting room that may or may not be read, you need your own record. The third way a symptom diary will help is by inviting you to connect your felt experience to language. The simple act of having to write it down will increase your body awareness, just like physical activity does. When we pay attention, we notice more and increase our personal wisdom of ourselves. If your gynecologic health feels great right now, track your gynecologic cycles or experiences for three months, then put the journal away. If anything changes in the future, you have a record of normal to come back to and compare. If you've noticed things are not quite right, or you've been adapting for too long, start tracking today and get scheduled with a gynecologist. They may need more data when you show up, but at least you've gotten started.

WE OWE NOTHING: BOUNDARIES FOR WOMB HEALING

I can't write about Black women healing without speaking to boundaries and recalibrating our threshold for saying no. This society does not deserve our energy, work, wisdom, or time, period. This does not mean we disengage from society; it means we are unapologetically laser-focused on intentional work only. Let your work be meaningful, and let your service be purposeful. Invest your efforts into work that replenishes your energy, not depletes it.* It takes time to start a physical movement practice, to journal your symptoms, and to attend therapy. To redirect our energy toward reconnecting with our wombs and ourselves, we simply need to be more unavailable. If it doesn't uplift you, it's a no. If it seems right but feels wrong, it's a no. Prioritize your time with yourself and your family—chosen or otherwise—first. Everyone else gets what may or may not be left over. Tell them no. Tell them I said so.

A CALL TO ACTION

We can reclaim the health of our wombs by refusing to suffer in silence, acknowledging when we're in pain, choosing action instead of neglecting that pain, and being aware of and mindful about our wombs when we're not pregnant. These are the steps to forge a path to a better quality of life for our wombs and a better gynecologic future for us all.

Step 1: Break the silence. Black women and all folks with a uterus must stop normalizing severe gynecologic bleeding, cramping, and pain. We must stop being silent in the face of debilitating pain and pressure from fibroids and heartbreaking infertility. Not speaking out on issues "down there" in an effort to deflect racist ste-

* I know many Black women are stuck in work that depletes them due to the insane economic inequities in our society. Those of us with more agency *must* do this boundary work, so we can be available to advocate for the political and economic policies that free us all.

reotypes (that we're hypersexual, for example) is killing us. We must normalize asking our mothers, aunties, sisters, and cousins about their gynecologic health and create a culture that is intolerant of suffering in silence. We must prioritize sharing information about our bodies, our symptoms, and our treatments with Black women in our families and friendship circles. And we must raise our children to think of this behavior as normal.

Step 2: We must acknowledge how our pursuit of achievement too often overshadows our commitment to not only our womb health but also our emotional, mental, and physical health. Our lives are not to be endured but to be enjoyed. The pressure of what life can bring—bad relationships, elder care, financial debt, and so on—can feel immense and impossible. We want to live fulfilling lives, not just physically subsist. Remember that affordable therapy is a powerful way to understand yourself and reclaim some agency in your life. Awareness and action are our keys to surviving the future.

Step 3: We must go to the doctor and seek help. I know what a tall order it is to ask Black women to trust doctors with their gynecologic health issues. But the very condition of being Black women in America means navigating a multitude of fraught spaces, and so this is not a new skill for us. We must use this skill to interface with our current medical system to access the information, treatments, and care that we deserve. In the next two chapters, I demystify the gynecologic visit and give you the tools needed to approach these spaces confidently.

Step 4: We must learn to demand respect from or change doctors if our symptoms are not taken seriously. In gynecology especially, your doctor must prioritize your quality of life. This book is written to arm you with both the biological understandings and symptomatic awareness to know when something is wrong and what must be investigated and improved. None of these conditions are simple, and neither are their solutions. In this sense, I am also arming us against the proliferation of non-evidence-based magical solutions that abounds online.

Step 5: We must demand more biomedical funding for and research into gynecologic conditions that severely affect Black women. That means advocating for more research funding, particularly when that funding will support the work of Black women scientists. These scientists often suffer from the same conditions they dedicate their careers to improving. In 2020, following the death of George Floyd, critics of medical education railed against the racist ideas still embedded in medical science. They also challenged the misogyny and misogynoir (the specific hatred, aversion to, or prejudice against Black women)* that allows most medical students to graduate with minimal knowledge or understanding of gynecologic health. In addition to mobilizing in support of funding and research, we must push for change in how doctors are trained.

The way we relate to our everyday, nonpregnant wombs is deeply connected to what's been passed down through generations in our families, how we value ourselves as Black women moving through the world. We can use our gynecologic care as a practical and powerful tool that helps us shift away from a strength that withstands suffering, silence, and pain to a strength that embraces our vulnerability and can demand better care from the larger world. We can become a sisterhood of Black women and a family of all Black folks with a uterus who reclaim a full, vibrant, healthy life. Womb Sisters.

* This term was coined by communications professor Moya Bailey, who came to the idea when studying old medical school textbooks for her dissertation work. Check out her Digital Apothecary lab at Northwestern University for more of her and her team's scholarship.

CHAPTER 9

WHAT DOES GREAT GYNECOLOGIC HEALTH LOOK LIKE?

By now, we've spent many pages walking through stories of what missing, inadequate, and disrespectful gynecologic care looks like. This was deliberate. Page after page, I sought to help you see our womb health plight for what it is—riddled with unnecessary suffering that we accept because we have been taught to do so. We must dream a new and better future of care for ourselves. I don't claim to have the complete vision of what optimal gynecologic care should look like, but I do have clear ideas that can guide us as we imagine together how best to get our health needs met. What follows is my perspective on the basics we deserve, informed by science and intuition, community knowledge, and esoteric expertise.

You should be able to count on my colleagues, members of the medical profession, to guide you in the communities where you live. Unfortunately, we know that not enough experts in women's health have the cultural humility necessary to offer us appropriate care. I hope this book inspires thousands of medical students to devote their careers to gynecology. I hope most of them are Black women, femmes, and gender-expansive people with a uterus. But even if that mass shift into gynecology happened today, as you are reading this book, it would still take five to ten years before you meet any of those converts in doctors' offices as board-certified gynecologists.

In the meantime, you need to become your own best advocate. We need to engage in gynecologic healthcare right now. In this chapter, I will explain to you what the general components of the gynecologic annual exam entail, with special attention to connections to other parts of your body and your well-being. I will pay particular attention to how we assess and diagnose causes of abnormal bleeding. So many of the conditions that Black women suffer from share this same symptom, and I'll help you to know how we use your history, your patterns, labs, and imaging tests to understand the root cause.

I think women can and should place gynecology at the center of how they assess their health. The gynecologic organs, and by proxy the reproductive health system, interact with most other health systems in the body. The reproductive health system can be a sensitive barometer of imbalance elsewhere and is central to our daily quality of life. This chapter will explain how each step in a complete annual gynecology visit touches on each aspect of gynecologic health, and therefore the rest of the body's health. By centering the womb and demanding quality care for it, you focus attention on the whole body.

THE ANNUAL GYNECOLOGIC VISIT AND EXAM

What follows is drawn from current published guidance for gynecologists and all physicians, nurse practitioners, and physicians' assistants who perform annual gynecology visits independently. There are also places where I respectfully disagree with the official guidance. I will note those instances and my rationale for you to make your own decisions. Mostly, I want you to be empowered with knowledge of what a complete evaluation looks like, so you and your provider are ready to make the most of it (and so you know if your provider has skipped over or rushed through important elements).

To begin, the overall guidance for doctors includes the following instructions for the setting and the tone of the visit.

- **The visit should take place in a private and relaxed setting.** The vast majority of the history (i.e., questions they ask you to understand you and any potential problems) should take place while you are fully dressed. There may be questions once the exam gets started that are prompted by your provider's findings, but otherwise, you should have your clothes on when going into detail about yourself. You will be more comfortable and less likely to speed through or omit important details. The same goes for after the exam, when you are discussing findings or next steps. After an exam, I always told my patients to get dressed before we talked, because they were likely to remember very little while sitting half-naked on my exam table.
- **The history-taking interview should happen alone with the patient and doctor.*** I respectfully disagree. If you know your doctor well, they know you well, and no surprises or important results are expected—fine. Otherwise, I recommend bringing a friend or family member, specifically a Womb Sister. There are many benefits to this: The extra person can remember details you forget about with respect to what is going on with you. They can ask questions you don't think of in the moment. They can be silent the whole time and just take in the vibe and communication skills of the doctor. A lot of us are naturally defensive and/or overly pleasing when dealing with physicians (including me in my own healthcare) because of the intense power dynamic. That can make it hard to get a read on whether the doctor was listening and responding to you well or not. Your Womb Sister can be a witness to help you sort that out, especially in an important or emotional visit. Finally, when hearing firsthand why a treatment or recommendation or test is

* I think this comes from a good place. Gynecologists and gynecologic oncologists know that sometimes we hear things that our patients have literally never told anyone else in their life. I respect that bond and always want to honor that sacred trust. And it makes me sad—because usually the secrecy is because of shame. And I want us to be done with that. Not everyone needs to know your business, but we should all have at least one person we can share our womb stories with. We deserve that kind of intimate community and support outside of the doctor's office.

important for you, a Womb Sister can help you stay accountable to the treatment plan, support any related needs (e.g., transportation, picking up meds), and be a great cheerleader. We don't have to do this alone. So here is permission to bring a friend.

- **Questions should go from open and straightforward to more sensitive and in-depth.** Not all healthcare providers are great communicators. If *you,* as the patient, want to dive right in to the juicy details of your bleeding woes, go for it. But it's normal and expected to warm up the conversation with basics about your health and your circumstances before we get to the nitty-gritty.
- **Assumptions should never be made about whether someone is sexually active or not, their sexual orientation, or their gender identity.** Throughout this book, you've already heard stories in which a healthcare provider's assumption that a Black woman was sexually active led to her pointed negative experiences, if not outright trauma. It is normal and expected for your physician to ask and confirm—and not assume—your gender identity, sexual orientation, and level of sexual activity.
- **A chaperone is present for the pelvic exam unless the patient specifically declines.** It's best practices to have a medical assistant, nurse, or other healthcare provider serve as a witness in case there is inappropriate behavior. This person might also hold your hand if you are indeed alone and need support for the exam. This role is designed to protect you, and having a chaperone should be opt-out, not opt-in. In other words, you shouldn't have to ask. Based on the clinic, they may allow your Womb Sister to be the official chaperone.

As mentioned, during a typical gynecologic health visit, your clinician will ask you a bunch of questions. We call that the *history*. A complete history in an annual gynecology exam is quite extensive and can take up at least half, if not more, of the visit. This is why physicians will often use a survey for you to pre-fill in the waiting room. This can definitely help with time efficiency, allowing them to skip over everything you marked normal and spend the most time on any issues or concerns. But patients aren't always clear on what the questions are asking or how to best respond, so it's good practice for your provider to confirm each piece of information live. This also helps jog your memory, in case you forget something important when quickly filling out a sheet. Whether your history is entirely verbal, or a mix of paperwork and a conversation, you want to be prepared to answer a lot of questions. Here are the most common and important elements of the history. Note that the order may vary, which is fine. The key is that no sections are missed.

- **Menstrual history**—We want to know it all, and you'll see why in the next section.
    - Includes: Age at your first cycle, your cycle length, and the number of days you typically bleed (including if it's all over the place).
- **Obstetrical (pregnancy) history**—Some conditions have different symptoms and different treatments depending on whether you have been pregnant before or not. For example, endometriosis is often much worse in those who have never been pregnant, and can improve for years after a pregnancy, only to relapse again. If you've never been diagnosed but have this pattern of symptoms, it's a strong clue for your gynecologist.
    - Includes: Total number of pregnancies, total number of births that happened between twenty and up to thirty-seven weeks, total number of miscarriages or abortions up to twenty weeks, total number of living children (specify if adopted children or surrogate born).
- **Sexual history**—This matters for so many reasons beyond whether or not you need contraception. I speak for any quality gynecologist when I say we truly do not judge you for whatever your answers are in this section. First, anyone who has worked as the gynecologist on call for the Emergency Department has

seen and heard it all.* Second, what you do or what you want to do in your sex life matters when we consider the impact of diagnoses and potential treatment plans. We can often work to balance all your considerations, but not if we don't know what they are.

 - Includes: Sexual orientation, sexual activity if present, number of typical or active sexual partners, frequency of sexual encounters. May include a request for specifics on type of sex depending on diagnostic or treatment needs.

- **Contraception history**—Tell us what you've used, how long ago you tried it, and why you loved or hated it. The biggest struggle we can have as gynecologists is that folks don't actually know what they took. The phrase *birth control pills* refers to literally *hundreds* of formulations, some with one active hormone, others with three or four. If you don't know, it's okay. Just know that it's unlikely you've "tried everything," and the more accurately you know your history, the better choices (and fewer failures) you and your gynecologists will have.
  - Includes: Type of contraception (pills, injections, IUDs, condoms, rhythm method, etc.); specific brand, name, or medication included; whether you took as recommended or prescribed; any side effects or struggles. Include any natural, or over-the-counter, or nontraditional practices or substances you take to avoid pregnancy.
- **Current symptoms (pelvic focused)**—Here is where that diary, journal, or log I suggested you keep comes in handy. As you go over what you've documented, make sure you also

* If only I had a different value system, I could tell stories for *days* about the things that happen in the dead of the night that become gynecologic problems in the Emergency Department. We'd have a whole different book and a good time. Unfortunately, I think these kinds of tales, especially told publicly by physicians, perpetuate the fear of judgment that keeps women and everyone who needs gynecologic care silent. This means we miss important aspects of their sexual health, and I can't contribute to that.

tell your gynecologist whether it is *your normal* or *a recent change*.

- Includes: Vaginal discharge/bleeding, vulvar or vaginal lesions, pelvic pain, abnormal bleeding, pressure, urinary or bowel issues (pelvic organ prolapse can feel as if your vagina/uterus/bladder is falling out, or can feel like a bulge), leaky urine, leaky stool / flatus (farts). What makes it better or worse? What pattern, if any, have you noticed? What have you tried, if anything? Are you concerned about it? If you are concerned, why?*

- **Infections and/or pelvic inflammatory disease history**
  - Includes: Any infections, such as yeast, gonorrhea, chlamydia, herpes, or HIV. Past treatments and whether they were successful. This is especially important if you've had recurrent infections that seem to be chronic.

- **Pap and HPV history**—The primary purpose of the Pap test is to screen for cervical cancer. Human papillomavirus (HPV) is a common sexually transmitted infection that can cause cervical cancer if left untreated. There is a huge amount of research on Pap testing intervals, risk factors, and how often and in what way to screen for cervical cancer. If you think the rules around Pap testing are confusing, you are in good company. Many healthcare providers would agree with you. How often you should get a Pap depends on your specific history. But because this is not something most of us are great about documenting, we often get the default screening plan. You may qualify for more or less screening based on your history.

* There are some folks who like to hold back here, especially with either what they have tried before or what another doctor has said. Perhaps they think this will allow them to have a clean slate with a new provider. In reality, you *are* biased by your prior experiences and that bias is actually *helpful* for us to know. If you've tried five things in the past and are frustrated, that may change what we initially recommend. If you had an experience before where someone didn't believe you or broke your trust, that helps us know where we stand. Give us the full picture.

- Includes: Any HPV vaccinations, last date and type of Pap testing, any history of abnormal results and what the result was, any prior treatment of abnormal cells ("freezing," LEEPs, biopsies, colposcopy), and those results as well. Your screening plan will then be made based on your history, prior testing, and current and future risk.

- **Other gynecologic history**—If it hasn't already been covered, this is where it can go. If your gynecologist knows about any prior gynecologic diagnoses, procedures, imaging, or surgeries, they are better equipped to help you while avoiding duplicate or unnecessary testing that costs money but doesn't give you more information.
  - Includes: Experiences with prior diagnosis of ovarian cysts, fibroids, infertility, endometriosis, polycystic ovary syndrome, and any other gynecologic or pelvic condition. We want to know when and how you received the diagnosis, how (or whether) it was treated, and if there is any active concern—and, if so, how you currently manage it. This is generally for things you have been diagnosed for in the past, though it is okay to bring up your suspicions if you don't have a confirmed diagnosis.

- **Gynecologic procedures and prior abdominal or pelvic surgery**—It's surprising how often this information is forgotten or missed! Take time to reflect on procedures and surgeries before your visit. If you desire intervention for any of your concerns, previous invasive procedures may have an impact on your treatment options moving forward.
  - Includes: Endometrial biopsies, cervical biopsies, laparoscopies, myomectomy, hysterectomy, salpingectomy (removal of tube), oophorectomy (removal of ovary), cystectomy (removal of cyst), and anything else that has happened down there. It helps if you have dates, the reason for the procedures, your recovery experience, and complications if there were any.

- **Screening for emotional and physical abuse, including intimate partner violence**—This should be a part of every annual exam. Gynecologists know that sometimes our exam room is the only place a woman who is experiencing a controlling partner is free to be alone. Expect these questions and understand that they are not due to any assumptions about how you look, dress, or behave. We know that abusive relationships happen at every socioeconomic level, in every community, and within all types of relationships. We ask everyone because we are a part of the safety net to help in these terrible situations.

As if this weren't already enough questions, there are usually more. We both need and want to know about any other medical diagnosis, especially mental health–related and chronic disease conditions. Your social context, like employment and your type of work and daily activities, is another factor that also matters. Understanding this helps to think about potential causes for new symptoms you may have, helps to prioritize treatment options when there are several on the table, and generally helps your gynecologist get to know your life better. There is usually also something called a *review of systems*—where a list of symptoms that represent other organ systems, like your heart, lungs, and kidneys, are also assessed. It is not infrequent that a gynecologic symptom can be a side effect of another primary issue going on elsewhere. This information can help connect all the dots.

THE PELVIC EXAM

Before we get into the specifics of what we are doing during a complete pelvic exam, I have to acknowledge this is another place where I respectfully disagree with the most recent guidance for gynecologists and other women's health providers. Some colleagues in my field have pushed to remove the pelvic exam as part of the routine annual exam, saving it for only when there are specific symptoms or concerns, to complete a Pap test,* to screen for sexually transmitted infections, or at the patient's request. I agree that a pelvic exam should certainly be done in response to concerning symptoms and to collect any necessary testing. But otherwise omitting the pelvic exam doesn't always make sense for Black women, who are too often the victims of neglect in the healthcare system. As an oncologist, I've seen too many cases in which the early signs of cancer were missed.

The first problem I see with skipping the regular pelvic exam is that it places too much of the burden on the patient to recognize what is abnormal and/or concerning and to report it in a manner the provider can be expected to take seriously. The second problem is that serious issues can be asymptomatic (no symptoms, no concerns) and only detected because of the pelvic exam. Asymptomatic lesions on the cervix or vaginal walls can be precancerous and removed before they become cancer. Fibroids are routinely underdiagnosed until they are too big to do anything but major surgery for symptom relief. An exam that reveals a uterus larger than expected may be the first clue of fibroids that are important to monitor. And though this next point may raise the eyebrows of my board-certified, evidenced-based colleagues, I think that detecting fibroids sooner can also give someone who is strongly oriented toward less conventional "treatments" a chance to try things out with lower stakes. Knowledge is power.

I do understand the rationale behind pulling back on automatic pelvic exams. We only want to do things in medicine that we know are beneficial and that limit harm. I believe a big reason the pelvic exam came under scrutiny was because of poor bedside manner and, frankly, abuse. When you have a field where male infertility specialists are impregnating unsuspecting patients with their own sperm,†

* Although with the new self-collect swab gaining FDA approval, Pap tests may be going away as a reason.

† You may have seen the documentaries *Our Father* or *Baby God,* but you may not know that this "fertility fraud" is not as uncommon as we might imagine. This happened in my own clinical department (he resigned and lost his medical license in the state). It is common enough for patient advocacy groups to be lobbying to make it an official crime punishable by jail time. Right now, in the majority of states, there are no legal consequences for this egregious abuse of trust.

you have a field with a major consent problem. I just don't believe that means we throw away the pelvic exam for everyone. Instead, it means we need better training, oversight, and accountability to ensure we're giving people with female reproductive organs the comprehensive care they deserve.

The pelvic exam does not need to be long and arduous to be complete. Gynecologists train for years to be able to distinguish normal variation from abnormal concerns. Here is what to expect during a pelvic exam. I've included some examples of anatomy we examine and potential concerns we can identify, but this is not exhaustive. My goal is to empower you, not try to teach medical school and clinical training in a few pages.

- **Explicit consent**—There should be zero doubt and clear affirmation that you consent to the pelvic exam. Because it has different parts—abdominal palpation, visual assessment, speculum exam, and bimanual exam—your provider can keep checking for consent at each phase or give you the overview, get consent, then proceed onward. It's okay if you consent to some parts of the exam and not others. We are supposed to work with you to figure out what you are comfortable with and to inform you what we may miss by skipping elements. The bottom line is that you decide.
- **Abdominal palpation**—We look and feel the abdominal wall down to the pelvic bone while you lie as flat as possible. We can detect signs of hernia or "asymptomatic" fibroids creating bulges. If you're experiencing pelvic pain, we can start narrowing down its causes.
- **Visually examine external anatomy**—We take a good look at all the parts down there we can see without any instruments.* These include the vulva, labia minora and majora, urethra, perineum, and anus. Many skin conditions can show up in these areas, including both noncancerous but serious (lichen sclero-

* I promise you we do *not* care if you shave, wax, or decorate that area the way you please. *At all.*

sus) and cancerous (vulvar cancer) conditions. We also look for signs of infection, urethral polyps, Bartholin's gland cysts, and painful fissures.

- **Visually examine internal anatomy**—We use the speculum to visually examine the vaginal walls, face of the cervix, and opening to the womb (cervical os). We look for lesions or signs of infection or inflammation on the vaginal walls, signs of changes related to low estrogen, such as color, elasticity, and fissures (associated with menopause or some medications), and cervical polyps or masses.
- **Examine the size, position, and mobility of the uterus**—We use our hands to do this. This is called the *bimanual exam* because we use both hands to do it. We place two fingers inside the vagina and one hand on the abdomen to feel the uterus. We are checking for enlargement, noting the tilt or position of the uterus (very important for any potential procedures), and mobility. Depending on someone's body size, we can detect potential pelvic masses and fibroids and get more information about sources of pain.* For bigger bodies, this part of the exam can be less informative, as even larger masses can be too small to feel through a thicker body wall.
- **Examine the back of the vagina and rectum**—It's called the *rectovaginal* exam, and it's done by placing one finger in the vagina and one in the rectum to assess the rectovaginal septum. This tissue can be thickened and nodular in endometriosis or have weakness or defects causing stool incontinence. This maneuver can also detect masses behind the uterus the we can't feel on the bimanual (vaginal-only) exam. In general, it is less routinely done unless there is a suspicion because of symptoms or other findings from previous parts of the exam that warrant

* I recently went to my gynecologist for increasing issues with my endometriosis. On my bimanual exam, she noticed a fullness on the left side and recommended we get an ultrasound. She was right. I had a large cyst on that side that was causing the weird pressure with bowel movements that I had been writing off. I had spent months trying to figure out what I was doing wrong with my diet. It wasn't my diet. Pelvic exams are useful.

more information. Gynecologic oncologists are more likely to do these exams—with consent—because of findings that can be related to cancerous disease in this area. Urogynecologists may also routinely include this exam for evaluation of the anal sphincter and prolapse.

In terms of making sure we receive good gynecologic care, there are a few more overarching things to consider, such as at what age to start visits. It is up to young people and their grown-ups to decide the right time for the first gynecologic visit. Remember that gynecology is much more than sex and contraception. General gynecologists, family medicine doctors, and pediatricians *should* all be excellent at teaching and caring for our young Black girls. However, too many women over the decades have shared with me story after story of traumatic initial gynecologic encounters, so I am going to err on the side of caution and recommend that teens see an adolescent gynecologist if they have access to one. These specialists are board certified for this specific kind of care and complete additional clinical training. With this type of clinician, I support the recommendations of starting at thirteen to fifteen years old.

In terms of my sisters out there who, for whatever reason, find the prospect of going to the gynecologist incredibly difficult, here are some ways to make it easier:

- Ask your gynecologist to talk through each step of the exam and what they are doing. They may need to think before giving you their thoughts and findings, but they can talk through what actions they are taking and ask permission on the way. If you prefer to be distracted by a random topic of conversation, music, or just getting lost in your own thoughts in silence, you can say that too.*
- Warmed instruments, especially the speculum, help a great deal. You can also ask the person conducting the exam for the

* I would ask my patients, "Do you want me to talk you through this, or do you want to be distracted?"

smallest size possible. Just know this may mean the first try is too small and we need to size up, as we have to move the speculum around to see all aspects of the vaginal walls. This may make the exam last a bit longer. There is a right size for everyone, and a patient gynecologist will find the right one with you.

- If the standard position (legs spread in the footrests while lying flat) is extremely triggering or impossible for you, there are alternatives: elevating the head of the bed thirty to forty-five degrees; putting one or both knees to chest; or even side-lying. Each of these is *less ideal* for everything we need to do, but much *better* than not having the exam at all.
- If your primary issue is chronic pelvic pain that may be worse during your periods, but also affects you greatly outside of your cycles, including and especially with sexual activity, I would recommend seeing a pelvic pain (or gyn pain) specialist if you can. Admittedly, these can be harder to find and may have long wait lists. In this case, see an excellent general gynecologist while you wait. But even one consultation with someone whose career is focused on gynecologic pain can change your life. These specialty gynecologists are also often trained minimally invasive surgeons and endometriosis specialists. At the very least, you want a gynecologist who lists pelvic pain as something they can and do treat. Conversely, there are gynecologists who want nothing to do with pelvic pain, and you need not have anything to do with them.
- Urogynecologists are our unsung heroes. They are included in the glossary as one of the many gynecologic subspecialists, but as an elder millennial with a post-pregnancy body, I had to give them a shout-out here. These wonderful surgeons treat all pelvic floor disorders, including prolapse, incontinence, and more. If one thing that keeps you away from the gynecologist is that you leak urine or stool or your vagina feels like it's bulging out—a urogynecologist is waiting eagerly to help you.

EVALUATING ABNORMAL BLEEDING

Because many Black women struggle with uterine bleeding, I want you to be informed about how we as gynecologists evaluate it. What follows is a deep dive into the evaluation of one common symptom, but I could just as easily invite you into an understanding of how a gynecologist should proceed if you complained of urinary incontinence, pelvic floor disorders, pelvic pain, or menstrual mood disorders. All symptoms deserve serious investigation.

There are two main parts to the process of figuring out abnormal bleeding: 1) hearing your story, and 2) conducting testing. Let's start with your story. Your gynecologist will ask you a number of questions from the above lists. When your responses indicate that your bleeding is concerning, we have some general ways of thinking about what is likely going on given the specifics you share.

Feature	Threshold for Concern	Notes
Frequency	Periods coming fewer than 24 (or 21) days apart (too frequent). OR periods coming more than 38 (or 35) days apart (too infrequent).	These definitions are based on the International Federation of Gynecology and Obstetrics. The US-based American College of Obstetricians and Gynecologists (ACOG) uses the numbers in parentheses.
Duration	Periods lasting more than 8 days (too long).	
Regularity	If the difference between your shortest cycle length	*Cycle length* refers here to the entire cycle. So, if your

	and your longest cycle length is more than 10 days, that is concerning.	period starts every 27 days, your cycle is 27 days. If that varies 10 or more days, that is irregular.
Flow Volume	Heavy, as reported by the patient.	See the text below this table for notes on this.
Intermenstrual Bleeding	Bleeding/spotting that happens between regular periods, noting if it is random or predictable.	If it is predictable and consistent, we further identify whether it happens in the early, mid-, or late cycle. This helps determine the cause and best treatment.
Unscheduled Bleeding	This is specific to those on hormonal medication and still bleeding unexpectedly. (Initial unscheduled bleeding is common when starting a new hormonal treatment.)	If present for longer than expected, it can mean a dose adjustment or medication change is needed. It does not have to be simply tolerated.

A few things to notice:

- If you have not tracked your bleeding and are guessing at many of these categories, your evaluation may be imprecise at the very onset. If you have any concerns about your bleeding, track your symptoms.* It is *critical* to your evaluation.

* I am of two minds about the use of digital tracking devices, like apps, for this. First, I understand how convenient they are and therefore much easier for many to stay consistent with logging their cycles. But I do fear our currently advancing digital surveillance state and the potential lack of privacy from data leaks or government oversight. This concerns me enough to err on the side of using physical journals.

- Heavy flow volume is patient-defined. That means it's up to *you* to know what is too much. It is not what your mother endured or whether your friends seem to think you are fine. You decide. As a reminder, *excessive menstrual blood loss* is defined as "when bleeding interferes with a woman's physical, social, emotional, and/or material quality of life." What quality of life do you deserve? To me, this is the most important question. However, if you are curious, these are some loose parameters of a "normal" flow based on a study where researchers actually measured the amount of blood collected in sanitary pads during a cycle and compared it to the reports from women about their cycle patterns. These normal parameters are used in common clinical references.

PARAMETERS OF A "NORMAL" FLOW
You change pads/tampons due to soaking them every 3 hours or MORE
You use fewer than 21 pads/tampons TOTAL for a cycle
You RARELY need to change your pad/tampon overnight due to soaking through it*
Any clots you pass are less than 1 inch in diameter†
You are not anemic by blood test

With this information, combined with knowledge of your medical conditions, any medications you may be taking and their effects, and your age, we then consider why this bleeding is happening. Very broadly, we can think of the causes as structural, physiological, or both. We use a handy acronym to keep all causes in mind: *PALM-COEIN*.

* Yes, I laughed out loud as well. Must be nice.

† See above. Many of us bleed too much. We don't have to.

This is an organizing framework endorsed by the International Federation of Gynecology and Obstetrics.

PALM is all things structural, meaning they are growths we can find using physical exam, imaging tests, cameras in the uterus, or biopsies. Each letter stands for a cause.

P—Polyps. These are usually noncancerous glandular tissues that grow in the endometrium.

A—Adenomyosis. This is when endometrial tissue grows in the muscle layer (myometrium, the middle wall)* of the uterus instead of the inner wall.

L—Leiomyoma. This is the medical term for fibroids.

M—Malignancy and hyperplasia. This is the medical term for cancer and pre-cancer.

COEIN are all things physiological, meaning they are changes in hormone levels, changes from medications, or that something unexpected is happening at the molecular or genetic level.

C—Coagulopathy. This refers to several blood conditions in which someone experiences an imbalance of blood-clotting and blood-thinning factors. When someone with such a condition bleeds, their bleeding lasts longer than it should.

O—Ovulatory dysfunction. This refers to a problem in the cycle of ovarian egg maturing and releasing. This can result from many causes like polycystic ovary syndrome, excess estrogen production, extreme diets that mimic starvation, and more.

E—Endometrial. This refers to a problem native to the endometrial tissue itself. For example, when women age past menopause, the endometrium naturally gets thinner and thinner, sometimes bleeding just because it's so fragile. We call this *atrophy.* Another example is *endometritis,* when there is an infection in the endometrial layer, causing bleeding from too much inflammation.

I—Iatrogenic. This is the fanciest term you can think of to refer to bleeding caused by doctors (or another healthcare provider) through a procedure, a medication, or supplement.

* Check out chapter 3, "The Basics," for a detailed explanation of the uterine anatomy.

N—Not yet classified. This is when we don't know, and often, we will use this designation while we are trying to figure it out, before all testing is complete. Just like in infertility evaluations, sometimes there is no smoking gun, and we use different treatment options in a trial-and-effect method until what works points us to what was wrong.

Each potential cause in the PALM-COEIN algorithm has many subcategories and requires nuance when applied to each individual. The goal here is not to make you a gynecologist overnight but to give you enough knowledge to know just how expansive the potential diagnoses are and a checklist to follow to ensure your doctor has considered each one.

TESTING

In addition to the detailed history-taking and story-making that offer clues as to why a patient is experiencing abnormal bleeding, there are tests and procedures that give us more information.

Pelvic ultrasound

The pelvic ultrasound takes the most accurate pictures possible of the uterus, tubes, and ovaries. It has two components—the abdominal scan and the transvaginal scan. The transvaginal scan in particular takes the best pictures of each layer of the uterus. It can detect fibroids, signs of adenomyosis, cysts in the ovaries and fallopian tubes, fluid in the endometrial cavity, and more.

Endometrial biopsy

If the endometrium (the inner wall of the uterus) is suspected as the source of the problem, a biopsy of that tissue can help give us more information. It answers the question: What is going on at the cellular level? For an endometrial biopsy, we use a slender flexible biopsy pipette that slides into the cervix and creates a mini vacuum in the uterus. The suction that is created brings endometrial tissue into the straw, so when we pull it back out, it has a sample of the endometrium. There are no sharp edges and no direct cutting. Most people will have very strong and painful cramps during and after a biopsy.* I strongly recommend asking for pain medication—at least a paracervical block. There is no need for any person to suffer through the cramps if they do not wish to do so.

Sonohystogram

This ultrasound-plus is sometimes also called a *saline-infusion sonohystogram,* or SIS. In addition to taking pictures of the uterus, this procedure places a small amount of saline in the uterine cavity to distend it, thus allowing better visualization of potential polyps or submucosal fibroids. This is often used in fertility evaluations to also assess how easily the saline fluid moves from the uterus through and out the tubes, which is important for natural conception to occur.

Hysteroscopy

In many ways, this is the gold standard of evaluating the endometrium because we get to look at it directly. In a hysteroscopy, a small camera is introduced through the cervix into the uterine cavity. We can see up close and personal what is going on. Hysteroscopy is often combined with treatment (e.g., removing the polyp you find or shaving down the fibroid sticking out into the cavity) to achieve diagnosis and treatment in one step. This requires anesthesia and can be done in a doctor's office with full-service sedation capabilities or, more often, in outpatient ambulatory surgery centers. The key is to work out a plan with your provider *ahead of time* to minimize your discomfort.

BLOOD TESTS / LAB STUDIES

Complete blood count (CBC)

This tests your level of red blood cells (and others) that circulate in your body. At a minimum, testing hemoglobin (or hematocrit)

* I have done hundreds of endometrial biopsies and can attest that some women feel nothing more than "a pinch," while others cramp for four days afterward. Humans truly vary, so focus on your own pain threshold and plan accordingly.

and platelet levels are a must. This is the test that defines clinical anemia.

Iron studies (ferritin)

There are several different ways you can measure iron, and I won't break them all down. To keep it brief, testing iron storage is maybe the most widely applicable. Iron storage is called *ferritin,* and low levels indicate iron deficiency.* Research has shown that a ferritin below 50 can cause symptoms that are improved with taking iron supplements. Below 20 is severe, and it is reasonable to start with IV iron transfusions and then transition to oral supplements.

Hormone testing

There are times when testing hormone levels is helpful. If ovulatory dysfunction is suspected, measuring progesterone *timed* to the expected mid-luteal phase, for example, can help to understand if and how ovulation is off. For older women who are not sure of their menopausal status, a follicle-stimulating hormone (FSH) test is accurate in determining whether or not lifetime ovulation has ended. Overall, there is currently not a broad, accurate test to predict exactly when menopause will occur before it happens. People's bodies vary widely, and just like the timing of when exactly a pregnant person will go into labor, we can estimate, but we cannot know for certain. However, after decades of research, we are making progress. In the Study of Women's Health Across the Nation (SWAN), a multiethnic, community-based study of the menopausal transition, over 1,500 women were tested and followed for years to track their menopausal transition. They looked at a number of hormones, including the anti-Müllerian hormone (AMH), using a specific sensitive test that detects extremely low levels.† Here's what they found—for women ages

* As a reminder, *iron deficiency* refers to having too little iron in your body for all the jobs it is supposed to perform. Iron-deficiency anemia is when the iron is so low that even its primary job—keeping your blood cells alive and delivering oxygen to your body—is also compromised. In iron-deficiency anemia, your red blood cell level is also low. See chapter 4, "Heavy Menstrual Bleeding," for more detailed discussion.

† "MenoCheck picoAMH ELISA" that detects down to 1.85 pg/mL (.00185 ng/mL).

forty-two to fifty-three, an AMH < 10 pg/mL meant menopause was highly likely in the next three years. If AMH was > 100 pg/mL, there was almost zero chance of menopause in the next twelve months. Because this study was funded by the National Institutes of Health with taxpayer dollars, the results are publicly available.

Hormonal testing should have a specific goal. Estrogen and progesterone fluctuate *wildly* during the normal-reproductive-age person's monthly cycles, and between people.* This is why gynecologists will rarely test either of these outside of specific cases, like the presence of a new ovarian tumor, infertility diagnostics, or evaluation of rare sex-based chromosomal conditions.

Other testing

Based on your history and symptoms, other labs may be needed. These include thyroid studies (TSH), coagulopathy labs, hemoglobin A1c and fasting blood glucose levels, and more.

There is a lot of information and discernment that goes into figuring out abnormal bleeding, and this is just one gynecologic symptom. I hope it's clear just how much assessment, evaluation, and treatment is available in a trained, caring gynecologist's office.

Gynecologic health is not and should never be considered optional. It's more than a TikTok reel, a "hormonal detox" program, or going vegan. I have only covered one symptom—abnormal uterine bleeding—here. This book doesn't even cover the ovaries, fallopian tubes, vulva, or vagina. Within abnormal bleeding, there are eighty-plus different potential causes when using broad overarching categories (like "cancer"), and more to count if we go in depth. This is why a board-certified gynecologist should be a part of your care team and certainly your treatment team.†

* See chapter 3, "The Basics," for the detailed overview of the ups and downs of these two hormones during the menstrual cycle.

† You can find the causes in appendix B at the back of the book. Feel free to make a copy and bring it with you if you want to follow along with your doctor's evaluation.

Achieving good gynecologic health means breaking our unhealthy relationship to suffering. The idea that women should bow our heads and endure uterine pain, bleeding, pressure, or cancer is an ever-useful tool of patriarchy. It keeps us physically distracted and drained. We can build entire spiritual disciplines around persevering despite our unhealthy wombs, but why must we suffer when we've been given the knowledge to heal?

Pursuing womb health means truly hearing your body when it screams out and attending to that pain rather than telling ourselves, "This is the way it's supposed to be." Sure, we can attune to and work in concert with the subtler messages our bodies send us. I am not opposed to *cycle syncing,** or arranging your work and activities around the ovarian phases of the cycle, for example. But we must better understand the distinction between normal and abnormal. Welcoming our blood is fine. But when we bleed too much, depleting the very oxygen meant to go to our brains and elsewhere, it's not enough to say, "This is my natural winter. I will just lie down." The fluctuations are not the problem. Fluctuating to the point of debilitation is the problem. The agency and power ultimately rest with you. You get to decide what pain, bleeding, pressure, and more you can and should manage on your own.

Be wary of oversimplification when the body is anything but simple. Though we gynecologists may have failed for years in communicating our science, medical research, and the rationale (and success!) behind many of our treatments, that doesn't mean they don't exist. I am incredibly enthused to see the changes brought by a wave of patient-centered care in gynecology. I am also excited to witness the boom in young, smart physicians opening up practices

* This refers to a growing movement for women to arrange daily life around the luteal and follicular ovarian phases of the cycle. I've always wondered why the focus wasn't around the endometrial phases (secretory, proliferative, and menstrual). Regardless, I love the way this idea encourages a strong connection with and awareness of how we feel. I don't love how it can inadvertently encourage women who need medical treatment to suffer through "natural" pain and bleeding. You can listen to your body and adjust your activities to not strain yourself. You can also recognize that your iron stores are too low, and bleeding less each month would go a long way to stopping the purge.

that are unapologetically focused on the conditions that affect Black women the most. I am proud of members of my profession for expressing more humility and for becoming more open to the idea that we don't know everything. But respectfully, we do know a great deal.

CHAPTER 10

MYTHS, VOCABULARY, AND POWER

MYTHS

As a gynecologic oncologist, I have seen women make life-altering decisions based on their belief in some enduring myths and misinformation. In some cases, these decisions ended up costing them their lives.

I met a woman with cervical cancer who was sure her problem was just too much "inflammation" and "unhealed trauma" of the womb. Her cervical cancer was caught early, when our cure rates with surgery and sometimes radiation are fantastic. She opted instead to put her all into alternative approaches. She started an "anti-cancer" diet, cut out sugar completely, and scoured the internet for "womb-cleansing" and "womb-healing" practices. She did ritual "steaming" and bought expensive yoni eggs. She removed stressful people from her life. When she came back after six months, she was sure her cancer would be regressing. You see, she had never felt better. All these changes—dietary, social, and physical habits—had transformed her daily life. She told me, though it was odd to say, that she was grateful for the cancer because it had given her permission to truly focus on herself and put her all into healing.

She was ready for her checkup exam. Her cancer had spread. She had gone from a stage I, where the cancer was only in the cervix, to a stage III, where it had spread to the tissues next to the uterus and to her lymph nodes. Now surgery was not an option. She needed chemotherapy, radiation, and immunotherapy. There was still a chance to cure her, but the path would be much, much harder. These were difficult facts for her to face, and I don't blame her for wanting a second opinion and wanting to hear a different answer.

She ultimately sought treatment at a center that markets themselves as being holistic and supportive of alternative therapies. They give much lower doses of chemotherapy than is required to kill cancer cells and add things like vitamin E infusions instead. The woman saw this as a great compromise and pursued the watered-down version of what she really needed. When I saw her again, a full year after her diagnosis, she was finally ready to take my "full recommendation." She felt her alternative therapies had worked somewhat, but acknowledged they were not curing her. In fact, her cancer was now beyond cure. The circuitous path to finally agreeing to the gold standard treatment for her condition meant that she missed out on the opportunity to benefit from the best options.

Ultimately, she did not survive her cancer. But before she died, I was happy to see her, as often as she liked, because I wanted to understand her. This woman wanted to live. She was not lazy. She was willing to change her entire life to heal her condition. To me, she was a victim of the long legacy of medical harm to Black bodies that creates earned distrust. She was also a victim of the irresponsible and predatory profit-driven myths that lead people down fruitless paths. Most of what she tried, especially initially, was either harmless or could have been helpful combined with evidence-based medical treatment. I think this is the reality *most* of the time.*

But there are some myths and practices that are simply not based in fact. They deliberately or unconsciously distort the truth and lead

* To be careful about disclosure, I've merged a few cases here and changed some details for anonymity. The crux—choosing alternative treatment instead of science—and missing the opportunity for cure was true in every case.

us astray in our pursuit of womb health. I have shared a tragic story here to illustrate the consequences of these unchecked myths. But these devastating outcomes can result from subtler starts, with reasonable-sounding logic and seemingly little negative effect. These myths and practices are insidious and are the reason why so many Black women turn away from treatments that can help.

When I see common myths around womb function, I do my best to tread carefully. I have no desire to demonize anyone seeking to support Black womb health. I am clear on the harms done by the field of gynecology through its propagation of racist and wrong beliefs about Black bodies. I also have never believed that all health wisdom is contained in medical textbooks or the Western biomedical framework.

In fact, I believe in integrating multiple streams of knowledge. I embrace both spirituality and scientific methodology. I have never understood these elements to be contradictory. To me, they are in harmony. I love the way astrology encourages me to consider different aspects of my personality, relationships, and work. I start each day by pulling a gratitude message from a card deck, and I feel certain the message that greets me is more than chance. I believe in God and the Divine and have felt the presence of energies that cannot be seen or understood.

And yet I need to dispel some ideas about womb health that lead to unnecessary suffering for people who have medical conditions that the biomedical system can help. The following list is not exhaustive, and you can blame me for any nuance missed. My hope is that most of this book has already busted myths by simply sharing through story, data, and science more than Black women typically get in their day-to-day gynecology encounters.

Myth: People with wombs should have a natural cycle every month to be healthy and keep things "clean."

Fact: If we are defining physical health as leading a full and thriving life free from unnecessary disease, then having a menstrual cycle every month is not necessary. As I mentioned in chapter 3, without intervention, everyone with a womb cycles much more today than we ever did in the past, because of the significant decline in how many pregnancies we have. If you would like to decrease your number of monthly cycles to match our ancestors via medications (e.g., hormonal birth control) instead of having ten kids, that is okay and not unhealthy.

Myth: The human body is perfectly designed and our problems and "dis-eases" come from external toxicity, toxins, and stress.

Fact: The human body is not "perfectly" designed without error. Actually, the way biology works is that our genetics are *just good enough* to keep most of us alive long enough to reproduce. Everything else is a bonus, evolutionarily speaking. Why are gynecologic diseases so common? Because, aside from cancer, they are rarely lethal. I don't believe that means we need to suffer from them without treatment.

Myth: This supplement / natural product / dietary change is the "true" cure for your womb, because here are countless women who have made it work for them.

Fact: Online, you may see a lot of success stories promoting "miracle cures" for things like endometriosis, adenomyosis, large fibroids, and other gynecologic conditions. But these results can be related to something called the *placebo effect*. The placebo effect is a well-known phenomenon in health studies and happens anywhere from 10 to 30 percent of the time based on the condition. If you believe something will help you, you will improve because your body just decides to get better. That is amazing! It also means the "cure" wasn't the herbal supplement, the magic shake, or the essential oil—it was you.*

In addition to the placebo effect, sometimes people are just not honest about other interventions they undertake simultaneously that contribute to their improvements. There is deceit in every industry, and there are several examples of wellness influencers who have faked their diagnosis or not disclosed that they had traditional treatment in addition to their magic supplement. I have rage for these people who exploit our natural desires to do well by our bodies.

In other cases, I think well-meaning folks simply don't realize

* This is why I meditate and visualize my healing all the time. I'm using *all* tools at my disposal.

that their natural, miracle cure is not for everyone, and they don't have the biomedical background to understand why that is the case. For example, there are forms of PCOS that are resistant to insulin and thus extremely sensitive to sugar intake. Reducing dietary sugar causes lower insulin levels, which results in less hormonal dysfunction, which ultimately leads to more normalized ovulatory cycles. If a person with PCOS had irregular heavy bleeding because of their abnormal ovulatory cycles, their radical sugar-free diet may work to regulate them. This does not mean a sugar-free diet will work for someone with fibroids, or polyps, or coagulopathy, or even PCOS that is not so insulin-sensitive. One size does not fit all. Nearly all the treatments I have discussed and recommended in these pages are options that have *outperformed the placebo effect* in well-documented clinical trials in the United States and around the world.* That is the threshold for scientific recommendation.

Myth: Hormones that come from outside of your body are not safe or natural. "Detoxing" from external hormones is the first step to good gynecologic health.

Fact: Hormones in birth control, IUDs, and menopausal hormone therapy are safe for most, though not all, people. But any time a study comes out showing an increased risk of this or that from "hormones" or "birth control," it takes off in the media like wildfire. I agree with Dr. Jen Gunter's take on this. Because patriarchal misogyny is rampant in our society, we are attracted to messages that demonize technologies that improve women's reproductive freedom, and those messages will always get the most media play. Did you know pregnancy increases the risk of breast cancer for the first five to ten years after birth for all folks over twenty-five years old? Probably not, because that is not a message that supports the widely held belief that women are born to suffer. Notice ways in which you may be predisposed to be distrustful of using the very molecules our bodies devised (hormones!) to treat hormonal conditions. Seems pretty natural to me.

* Surgical studies generally compare one procedure to another, as placebo surgery is quite difficult to pull off and would put people under anesthesia risk without any benefit.

Myth: I tried hormones and they didn't work for me. I can't tolerate them.

Fact: "Hormones" is just about as generic as saying "chemotherapy." There are literally hundreds of different hormones, in different formulations, at different doses, that interact with different bodies differently. Having a bad reaction to one medication does not mean that you must avoid all hormones for life. A great gynecologist can walk you through this so you don't go untreated for menorrhagia, fibroids, endometriosis, or the early signs of uterine cancer (hyperplasia).

Myth: Pharmaceutical companies and by extension doctors work together to demonize alternative medicine to keep medical profits high.

Fact: There is not an organized conspiracy to suppress effective "natural" treatments in gynecology. That would imply there is a high level of pharmaceutical interest in women's health! As I detailed in chapter 2, "Origins," our primary problem is not conspiracy in women's health research—it's neglect. For many years, I would hear anecdotes from patients about how changing their diets improved their period pain. I could relate. When I decreased my intake of fried foods and dairy, my menstrual pain lessened. This also happened after I had my first child, and pregnancy is known to decrease endometriosis symptoms. If I go on vacation and eat a lot of fried fish and mac 'n' cheese, I will be cramping the next week. This information is not being suppressed. In fact, how the gut and the microbiome impact gynecologic conditions is an active area of research. Scientists are getting into the details of bacteria, genetics, food sources, and outcomes to better understand this and develop new recommendations and treatments. But because the threshold for scientific evidence to make medical recommendations is so high, it takes time to understand and clarify what the data shows. In the meantime, if your dietary changes aren't giving you the results you want, it's not a failure to consider medical treatment.

Myth: A women's health social media influencer with a large following is trustworthy.*

* One of the reasons it took me years to share anything health-related online despite being a scientist and expert in the field was because of how often such power and privilege is abused. Especially online, we want things to be simple and straight-

Fact: If you have a gynecologic diagnosis—endometriosis, symptomatic fibroids, or heavy bleeding, for example—and/or if you have a family history of breast or gynecologic cancer, please do not take your gynecologic advice from untrained social media influencers. Talk to a board-certified gynecologist or subspecialist in person. Get a real consult.

Myth: "Do your research" means watch YouTube videos or scroll websites selling alternative treatments.

Fact: If you choose to go with any kind of holistic treatment, especially one that suggests alternative supplements or other interventions beyond lifestyle or dietary changes, do this first: Look up the treatments on WebMD or the patient version of UpToDate so you can see if any supportive scientific evidence exists. Don't trust the testimonials. Talk to people who have tried the method directly (not via a testimonial) so you can clearly compare things like your illness severity, other conditions, and life circumstances with theirs. Be sure to ask about anything else they were doing alongside the nontraditional treatment. It is very common for people to highlight the "alternative" treatment they do, while not mentioning more traditional medical therapies they are *also* doing or did. Unfortunately, we see this a lot in endometriosis, fibroids, and gynecologic cancers. Set specific goals of what you want to see improve for yourself, and commit to tracking that. Keep a diary and set a timeline to reassess. As we've discussed, things can worsen while we are not paying attention. It's okay to stop an alternative therapy if it's not working.*

---

forward. Yet nothing about Black women and womb health is. So, I decided to write this book in addition to the content I share online.

* I hate the phrase *do your research*. As a researcher, I spent years in medical training, then two additional years full-time in graduate school to learn how to design and execute quality studies. It takes me considerable time and attention to read a study, in its native scientific language, to understand exactly how it was done to determine if the results are sound or not. There are many times when some aspects of the study are reasonable but others are not. In other words, "do your research" takes training to understand what quality scientific research is and whether or not a study makes sense or can be applied to you.

As I detailed in chapter 8, gynecologic or womb health is much more than physical. The physical doesn't even matter if we don't know our family stories, can't connect to our emotions, and can't feel our own bodies. Gynecologic health is by nature multidisciplinary and multifaceted because of all the ways having a womb impacts your life in this society. Seek healing in all ways that resonate with you, but keep science, facts, and evidence in the mix. Please.

VOCABULARY

Vocabulary matters. In the stories you read in this book, we saw the power of vocabulary for Black women interacting with the gynecologic healthcare system. Dr. Whitney Robinson had to use the words *breakthrough bleeding* to get through the scheduling wall of her own gynecologist's office. Dr. Mya Roberson had to diagnose herself, naming "I have endometriosis" to finally get a referral to an off-campus specialist. It wasn't until Dr. Rose essentially said, "I can't breathe," that someone finally imaged her expanding uterus. Words matter. As one of my favorite podcast hosts Crissle West of *The Read* says, "Words Mean Things."

The burden should not be on Black women to have the right words to unlock medical curiosity, empathy, and action. But the current world we live in is not one where Black women experience the privilege of being legible to their doctors by default. Here are words and phrases you can use as communication tools to more effectively reach your clinician.

When describing your symptoms:

"This is a persistent change from my baseline. This is not my normal."

This indicates that something has changed and it's lasted long enough to investigate. If you've kept a diary, you can add the specific timeline.

"Because of {symptom}, I am unable to do basic activities of daily living."

For symptoms that don't kill or outwardly maim you, the medical threshold for intervention is often when you can no longer do regular or routine activities. If you used to be able to complete a regular workday, and now you only make it half a day before you are too tired to continue—that is *severe fatigue* that interferes with your daily activities.

"For me to {insert activity}, I now have to do {insert adaptation}."

For most of us, we don't stop; we adapt. For an outside observer, it may appear that we don't have "deficits," because we are still getting it done. We need to get comfortable with exposing these adaptations that often speak to the severity of our symptoms. For example, "For me to not have a bleeding accident on a long flight, I have to wear three pads and an adult diaper."

When discussing the options in diagnosis and treatment:

"What is the differential diagnosis?"

This may sound like a mouthful, but if you don't feel like you're having an expansive conversation with your doctor, this question appeals directly to how we are trained. The *differential diagnosis* is the list of all possible causes your symptom may have (within reason). An example of a differential is the PALM-COEIN list for abnormal bleeding.* If you understand this, you can then understand the how and why behind each diagnostic or treatment step your doctor recommends.

"What makes this the best {diagnosis or treatment} option, in your opinion? What information will it tell us?"

I thought about this phrasing for a while. Doctors have opinions—a lot of them. Some are born of our training and some of our experience practicing and others just from our lives. Your doctor may have a reason to recommend a step to you after assuming your preferences inaccurately. This question can uncover those assumptions so you can be sure they align with what you really want.

"How will we know whether {treatment} is working? When do we check in again?"

So many times, I see a Black woman seek gynecologic care, have one perfunctory visit with one treatment offered, and never go back. If the symptoms don't improve, there was no plan. This question ensures you are clear on the timeline and the follow-up plan. For ex-

* See chapter 9 for the breakdown of PALM-COEIN.

ample, some treatments can take three months before you see improvement, but the positive effect will last for five years. If you don't know that up front, you might stop before the treatment has a real chance to work.

Symptom vocabulary specific to gynecology

Breakthrough bleeding—You have regular periods but bleed in between cycles.

Irregular cycles—Your cycles are not predictable. You could not bet on when they come and how long they last. Often a sign of ovulatory dysfunction.

Bulk symptoms—This refers to all the ways an enlarged uterus creates pressure and discomfort. It can include feeling pressure on your bladder or colon, frequent urination (that is a change from baseline!), constipation that is persistent no matter where you are in your cycle, or a growing waistline where you may even feel a firm mass (your uterus) underneath.

Postmenopausal bleeding—The classic definition includes any blood discharge, spotting, bleeding, or clotting that happens in the menopausal years, which means after at least twelve months with no bleeding at all. For Black women, I will hear that "I never stopped bleeding, but it got lighter for a while, then picked back up." If this is you or a loved one, call it *postmenopausal bleeding* so you can get in and get evaluated.

A note for healthcare providers

If you have gotten this far, you will have noticed how often Black women suffer in plain sight in the healthcare system, despite attending the doctors' visits that should help them. I want to offer some vocabulary for my colleagues as well, especially as it relates to caring for Black women.

1. Assume a curious posture. Remove the burden of symptom disclosure from Black women. Ask about bleeding, pain, fatigue, and pressure symptoms directly and explicitly. Circle back and ask again.

2. Subjective words like *heavy, bothersome, severe,* and the like have a different threshold for Black women, because our lived experience too often tells us suffering is normal. Move away from the subjective and ask instead about impact on daily activities and adjustments to daily life.
3. In medicine, we have a bias that if something has been going on a long time—say, for years—it must not be that bad, because the person is still functioning. We need to remove this bias completely when dealing with Black women. The length of symptoms does not indicate a lack of severity but rather the strength of the person who has endured for so long. Move accordingly.
4. Be flexible and proactive in follow-up and err on checking in sooner rather than later. A Black woman in your office is already making a huge leap of faith to discuss her womb with you. Visits aren't only for test results. They are for building trust too. Check in earlier.
5. Ask this question: *Are you happy with your gynecologic health (or your periods, or your {insert gyn symptoms}) or would you like it to be better?* Normalize this question and make space for the response. We have incredible tools to alleviate suffering in people's everyday lives, but we cannot use them if we do not ask.
6. *Not yet,* or *not now,* or *I'm not sure* is not a permanent *no.* We are led to believe through our training and our society that the decades of schooling and hardship required to become an independently practicing physician mean people should do what we say the first time we say it. Humans don't work that way, and Black women would have gotten nowhere in life if we did that. You demonstrate trustworthiness by not being offended or frustrated by a no and instead using it as a bridge to understand your patient better. Instead of being offended or frustrated when a patient says no to something you are clear would help them, try this: *"Thank you for being honest with me. I'm glad you trust me enough to say no. Can we revisit this again in X {days, weeks, months}? I just want to be sure you are getting the best care possible."*

POWER

Ultimately, all this talk of myths and vocabulary is about claiming our power. I believe power exists in us all, to a degree that is often underutilized. In my life, I have consistently outperformed expectations, landed in places that were theoretically not open for me, and reached "impossible" goals. I agree with the saying "Luck is preparation meeting opportunities." I know how hard I work and what it means to stay ready. And I know that everything I have achieved is also because I saw it first for myself. I am not surprised, because I dreamed it. I am prepared because I took those dreams seriously.

The goal for Black women and gynecologic health should be a shared, overarching, transformational dream. Gynecologists everywhere. Easy and effective treatments for fibroids, endometriosis, heavy periods, and uterine cancer. No more needless suffering. Our power comes from knowing what we deserve and demanding it.

On our way to achieving that collective dream, you'll need to advocate for your own gynecologic health. The care you receive should feel tailored to your history, the setup of your life, and your short- and long-term goals. A gynecologic new patient appointment that doesn't start with a detailed history is a red flag. More than anyone else, Black women need individualized gynecologic care. Our context is unique, and our bodies exist, struggle, strain, and bleed in this context. Gynecologic treatment should be driven by patient preferences, and your preferences are driven by your context. How can you receive a recommendation you are likely to feel good about if your doctor doesn't know your preferences?

Your gynecologic healthcare should feel warm and empathetic. We climb significant hurdles to get to a place where we can discuss our womb health openly and securely without judgment or shame. Quality gynecologic healthcare requires detailed and accurate disclosure of symptoms. The medical establishment has not earned this level of honesty from Black women. If you are going to take a leap of faith, you deserve to do it with a warm and empathetic gynecologist. Find a provider who knows how to elicit your story and how to talk to Black women with respect. Find a provider who can draw you all the diagrams you may want and who wants to earn your trust. Bedside manner, intelligence, and excellent clinical skills do not have to be mutually exclusive.

You should hold the same standard for your gynecologic health-care providers that you hold for romantic partners. *What?!* Yes, I said it. I invoke this metaphor intentionally. Gynecologists differ just like potential boyfriends, girlfriends, or they-friends. Just because you've had one or more bad experiences doesn't mean all gynecologists are terrible. Similarly, gynecologists' communication styles and approaches vary like those of potential significant others. You might just not connect with the vibe, and that's reason enough to keep looking. You need a gynecologic health home that feels comfortable for all the reasons mentioned. You must be able to share everything, and you can't do that if you're on the defensive as you walk in the door.

Gynecologists sometimes have to tell you things you don't want to hear, just like any true friend would. If your goal is to find a doctor who never delivers unwelcome news, you will not have a partner in health; instead, you will have someone whose aim is to keep you happy regardless of your health. If you're unsure whether the information you are receiving is poor quality and disrespectful, or good quality but hard to accept, bring a Womb Sister to a follow-up visit for a second opinion. You have the power to move on from a doctor who just isn't right for you.

We do have agency and power to demand this quality of care. I know Black women are often asked to fight for others, because our voice and conviction are so powerful. I want us to use that power for ourselves, in service of our everyday womb health. We are moving from a position of terrible strength to one of confident power. We have what we need. Let's go.

A Love Letter to Black Women

Dear Sister,

We are not broken and we are not destined to suffer. We can recognize the multigenerational inheritance of quiet endurance, of a regal resilience, and still decide we can and will live differently. Even if you have not experienced any of the many symptoms detailed in this book, you know a Black woman who has—your mother, auntie, cousin, daughter, friend, co-worker. You may have seen your whole secret struggle laid bare in these pages and need to grieve for the ways you were taught to live your own terrible strength. I write this letter to us, for us. I want to give you permission to create a compassionate and healthy relationship to your womb health. I want to share with you the responsibility we have to hold one another's womb health in high priority. And I want to help you release the need to be hyperfunctional at the expense of your body and your well-being. Sisters, self-neglect is not a virtue and your brilliance is not a call to do and take on more than is healthy for you to endure. I write to help you honor your vulnerability, to gently hold your fragility, and to refuse the standards of a world that can see and hold neither.

Let us declare these truths, together, now.

—Womb suffering is not our birthright.

—Our pain is real and our healing is possible.

—We deserve to walk, run, laugh, and live with a full tank of blood, like our bodies were designed to have.

—We are our Sisters' Keepers. Sharing womb stories and supporting one another's womb health is an intimate friendship we can all be a part of.

To the Black girls and young women who are aspiring gynecologists, I want you to know that the practice of gynecology is your birthright and legacy. I want you to know that your people, connected to you by DNA, a common racialized experience, or both, are the bodies upon whom gynecology was built. Pursuing this important, complicated, and powerful field of study is your lane entirely. The blood of your mothers and their mothers and their mothers and their mothers nourished the roots of biomedical science. Stand tall and in honor of our incredible matrilineal legacy. Study, stay focused, don't let challenges knock you off your path, and persevere in service of the Black womb.

To the doulas, womb-wellness practitioners, herbalists, naturopaths, and all others seeking to do right and well by Black people and our wombs, I hope you have found welcome, respect, and valuable information in these pages. I thank you for treating Black women as more than diseases to fix or bodies to learn upon. I hope I have succeeded in gently pushing against some ideas that I believe were born with the right intention but have become blanket solutions that simply do not serve us all well. I hope you found within these pages extra tools to add to your approach of womb wellness, stripped from the oppressive origin they may have. I hope above all we share the same love and awe of the Black body and the womb, and move with a commitment to benefit from all we have learned scientifically and otherwise. Thank you—we need you.

To little Kemi, who was told she was too much—too angry, too talkative, too sensitive, too dark, too ugly, too loud, and even, hilariously, too hardworking—I thank you for sticking around, waiting patiently for me to embrace you to your fullest. I am so grateful my attempts to change and mold you were never successful for very long. This book is all too much, and it is beautiful. Thank you.

To my grandmother Omotayo, and to the women whose names I don't know, who came before her for thousands of years, I thank you for the life you led that ultimately created mine. I thank you for the wisdom you imbued in me before I could recognize what it was. Your name signified the coming of joy, and I hope this book, this offering, brings just that to you, to your daughter, to me, to my daughter, and to the thousands of years of our line to follow.

Acknowledgments

Writing this book has been an exciting, vulnerable, and intensely rewarding experience. I am grateful to God for trusting me with this life. I am grateful to you, readers, for taking the time to join this part of the journey.

Whitney, Mya, "Rose," and Ms. Barbara—thank you for your trust in me and your bravery in telling the stories that are so often silenced. Every time I sat with you, your words changed me in some way, and now they will change the world. Thank you.

I am thankful to all the women I've had the honor of calling my patients. The ups and downs of your health journeys, the tears and the relief, the fear and the joy—all the moments mattered. Thank you for your trust and for teaching me too. For children, spouses, and friends of the women who didn't make it, your loved one mattered and their memory stays with me.

I have gratitude for so many people: Ms. Bridgette Hempstead, you have passed but are not forgotten. Thank you for receiving me with open arms, mothering me, guiding me, and being my friend. Adrienne, Margie, and the entire ECANA community—I love you, I thank you, and I am so proud of the work you carry on. To my incredible team at the GRACE Center—Julianna, Nadia, Patrice, Leah, Beza, and Adrienne—thank you for bringing your heart to our science and your dedication to our mission. You all are the cream of the crop!

The research I present here is a consequence of so many important times someone said "yes." Dr. Barbara Goff met me as an ambitious gynecologic oncology trainee and recruited me to the University of Washington. She said yes to my unique career path when most would have said no. Thank you for your trust, your support, and your guidance. We need more leaders like you. Dr. Elizabeth Swisher, thank you for being my ultimate cheerleader, sponsor, mentor, and friend. Dr. Charles Thomas, our first talk changed my life. To the small-but-mighty group chat of Black women gynecologic oncologists who paved the way and those coming after me, where would we be without one another? Thank you for your community. To all of my stellar clinical teachers and colleagues, there are many stories in this book of healthcare gone wrong, yet everything I learned about how to be a skilled, discerning, and compassionate surgeon came from you. Thank you all for holding me to the highest standards and giving me a platform to do my best. "My" perspective is only mine insomuch that I have inhaled the writings of brilliant Black women scholars who opened my eyes to dimensions of race, gender, and health far beyond what medicine would give me: Chandra Ford, Brittney Cooper, Angela Davis, Deirdre Cooper Owens, Tressie McMillan Cottom, Karen Scott, Dorothy Roberts, Camara Jones, and Chandra Prescod-Weinstein. Thank you. Scientific research is a team sport. To my scientific collaborators and mentors—Dr. Whitney Robinson, Dr. Erica Marsh, Dr. Scott Ramsey, Bryan Comstock, Dr. Ronit Katz, Dr. Danielle Lavallee, Dr. Erika Wolff, Dr. Rosana Risques, Sarah Monsell, Dr. Mindy Pike, Sarah Romano, and Dr. Kristin McCowan—thank you for being smart, committed, skilled, *and* kind.

Respectfully, my life squad is unmatched. To Liz, Ali, Monique, Karen M., and Shirlene—you have held me down in the valleys and celebrated loudly with me at the peaks. I treasure you. Thank you. Jereshia, my life would be so much smaller, less colorful, and less joyful had we never met. Thank you for changing my life. KD Coach

Community!!! Thank you for being on this ride with me, listening to updates years before there was any book to purchase or read, and reminding me every day that dreaming big is always worth it. Y'all got next.

Nikole Gianopoulos, you are a one of one. Thank you for holding me down, keeping me organized, and staying one step ahead of the chaos of this multi-passionate big dreamer's life. Working with you is an absolute delight.

As a seasoned scientific writer, I embraced the opportunity to be a learner again with the style, pacing, and tone of this book. Thank you to Dani McClain, my careful and insightful development editor, who knew the perfect balance of praise and redlining to help me shape these pages. Thanks to Jane Jones, a fantastic book coach, who helped me stay organized, stay sane, and plan the best strategic breaks. To my clinical readers—Dr. Monique Farrow, Dr. Kimberly Kho, Dr. Sarah Temkin, and Dr. Sara Whetstone—thank you for bringing your eye to this work. The disease chapters are better because of you. Thank you, David Walters. Your copyediting and fact-checking gave me the last confidence boost I needed to put this work out in the world. Invaluable. Thank you!

Thank you to my amazing literary agent, Tanya McKinnon, who said *tell me everything*—then listened. You took my unorganized ideas and helped me mold the full vision of this book. You expanded what I thought was possible and then showed me what it looked like to really go after it. You are exceptional, thank you.

Jamia Wilson, there are no finer hands for a passionate debut author to be in but yours. *Editor* is far too small a word to encompass your role. Thank you for the "gentle excavation," the clear guidance, and your above-and-beyond commitment to my book. We know who brought us together, and I hope that I have made her proud.

And big thanks to Diana Baroni and Marnie Cochran for welcoming me into the Harmony fold, and Miriam Khanukaev, Julia Diaz-Young, Monica Brown, Hannah Dirgins, Theresa Zoro, and everyone at Team Harmony for working so hard on this book—thank you!

To my mother, Lola Oni-George, for giving me life, loving me, and never letting go. I am grateful for the relationship we have made together today. Leke, I'm so glad we choose to be family. Thank you to you and Keyona for the laughs, motivation, and real talk. There were treasured individuals whose love kept me whole when I was young and needed it most: To Karen and Leanne Shutt, who were gentle with me when I was small and all sharp edges; Kane and Michael Gathings and Liz McKenney, who provided me safe harbor in rough seas; and Neal and Nanci Solomon, whose kind energy helped me see myself in a different light. Thank you.

To Rick and Gayle Doll, the grandparent GOATs—thank you for everything. The list is long.

Simon and Amaya—I love you both fiercely and I always will. Thank you for making me laugh, giving the best hugs, and beating me in Play Nine every . . . single . . . time. You are both extraordinarily good and wonderful people, and I feel so lucky to be your mom.

Jake—you are my forever. Your foundation frees me to soar. I love you. Thank you.

Appendix A: A Primer on Finding Quality Gynecologic and Gynecologic Oncologic Physicians

Without fail, every few weeks, a Black woman messages me asking how to find a good gynecologist or gynecologic oncologist. I know these messages are not about how to use Google or decipher patient satisfaction ratings online. These Black women reach out to me because they already know that a string of accolades is no guarantee of good care for the Black body. They reach out to me for a deeper kind of referral. They are asking me for help in finding a clinician they can trust with their Black body. In this supplemental chapter, I will share what my Black physician colleagues and I do when we need to find a doctor for ourselves, our friends, or our family members. My goal is to democratize this knowledge for Black women because healthcare can be a treacherous environment for us.

Best practices for finding a quality gynecologist or gynecologic cancer specialist:

LOCAL-KNOWLEDGE REFERRAL

If you have a good relationship with a current physician, regardless of their specialty, ask them for a recommendation from their personal network. This is how doctors choose what doctor they will see. We don't google, and we don't look at star ratings. We start with the colleagues we know and often trained beside and ask them to identify someone whose work they respect in the specialty we need. Alternatively, we may know someone at the institution where we or a loved one are to be treated, and we ask the same questions. "My sister-in-law needs a hysterectomy for a large uterus, done at your hospital. Can you please find out who is the best referral for this kind of case?" In other words, we always try to access skills-based, local, and direct knowledge recommendations.

BEDSIDE MANNER

In medical school and clinical training, you realize that doctors' interpersonal skills vary greatly and are not always correlated with diagnostic or procedural talents. In other words, there are some awkward, distant doctors who are fantastic surgeons, and some warm and charismatic doctors who are deeply uninformed on the latest medical knowledge and practices. There are introverted doctors who are quiet and shy but smart and incredibly attentive. And yes, of course, there are plenty with both: great interpersonal skills and fantastic clinical acumen. Be sure to distinguish the two, and bring a Womb Sister to help you assess. A renowned provider who treats you poorly by not giving you basic respect (listening to you when you speak, believing your symptoms, answering your questions) is not worth any degree of clinical skill. Not everyone agrees with me here, but I stand by this. No matter how skilled they are, if your doctor can't treat you like a functioning and capable adult, then the care isn't worth it. They will not treat you as an equal in the plan for your own care and your own treatment. When it comes to your health, don't ignore your gut instincts, and don't be afraid to voice your concerns directly to your doctor.

Great doctors tell you up front what they do and don't know and why.

As you've read, there is still a great deal we don't know about gynecologic disease and gynecologic health. Yet there is much we can do to alleviate your suffering and prevent life-threatening complications. Look for a doctor who can explain their thinking to you and isn't shy about telling you why they do or don't know the answer to your questions. Many times, I've had to say words like, "I don't know why this caused side effects in you and not in other people, because, sadly, we just don't have a lot of research in this area. What I do know is that this side effect is not permanent and your symptoms will improve once we stop the medication. Because you are benefiting from the medication, I recommend you continue for three more weeks and then we stop. What do you think?" The last sentence is critical. That is where I invite my patient to be a participant in her own healing and not a passive vessel for my prescriptions. As a side note, tread carefully with any clinical provider, from any medical, wellness, or health tradition, who has an answer for everything and knows all.

SPECIALIZED CARE FOR RARE CONDITIONS

If you need a specialty procedure or have a rare condition, consider searching for medical centers with active clinical trials or who have active, accredited training programs in your area of need.

These institutions will be most up-to-date on available treatments, operate within a culture of multidisciplinary input to care, and are required to have a certain level of volume and experience with these procedures to maintain an accredited training program.

Find advocacy groups for Black women to seek out someone who has or had your condition. These can be great sources of knowledge for doctor referrals, and often you can hear about different styles and decide who may work best for you. These folks can be an invaluable resource in sharing their experiences and knowledge. These groups also often work hard to share diagnostic and treatment information in easy-to-understand terms, and can have downloadable templates and educational videos that help prepare you to get the most out of your doctors' visits.*

* ECANA's website has excellent resources for this (ecanawomen.org), and you can find more information at the Gynecologic Research and Cancer Equity (GRACE) Center (www.gracecenteruw.com).

Appendix B: 83 Potential Causes of Abnormal Female Genital Bleeding*

Vulva	Atrophy / ulceration Skin tags Lichen sclerosis Fissure or tear Polyp Sebaceous cyst Condyloma Urethral polyp / mass Angiokeratoma Infection Dermatitis Cancer Trauma
Vagina	Atrophic vaginitis Bacterial vaginosis Sexually transmitted infections Contact dermatitis Polyp Gartner duct cyst Adenosis Cancer Fissure Trauma

Cervix	Inflammation (cervicitis) Dysplasia Polyp or mass (benign) Polyp or mass (cancerous) Trauma Infection
Uterus (womb)	Endometritis Hyperplasia Atrophy Endometrial polyps Submucosal fibroids Adenomyosis Arteriovenous (AV) malformation Cancer (adenocarcinoma) Cancer (sarcoma) Menstrual cycle dysfunction Pregnancy related Adjusting to new hormonal medication† C-section scar defect
Ovary / fallopian tube	Hormonally active ovarian cyst Ovarian cancer Fallopian tube cancer Pelvic inflammatory disease
Nonhormonal medication	Anticoagulants Thyroid medication Corticosteroids Phenytoin Antipsychotic drugs
Trauma	Penetrative sexual intercourse Sexual abuse Foreign bodies Misplaced IUD Pelvic blunt force trauma Straddle injury (e.g., bike seat)

Bleeding that is mistaken as vaginal or vulvar but is not	Urethral lesions Bladder cancer Bladder infections Colon cancer Inflammatory bowel disease Hemorrhoids Anal fissures Anal polyps or masses
Systemic conditions that can have abnormal genital bleeding patterns	Crohn's disease Behçet syndrome Lichen planus Lymphoma Thyroid disease Liver disease (advanced) Cushing syndrome Kidney disease Smoking Thrombocytopenia or platelet dysfunction Von Willebrand disease Coagulation factor deficiency Excessive exercise Emotional or physical stress Anorexia / bulimia Primary ovarian insufficiency Alcohol or other drug abuse Diabetes mellitus

Adapted from Kaunitz, A. Abnormal uterine bleeding in nonpregnant reproductive-age patients: Terminology, evaluation, and approach to diagnosis. In: UpToDate, Connor RF (Ed), Wolters Kluwer. (Accessed on April 10, 2025.)

* These are the common causes. I have not included very rare things like Stevens-Johnson syndrome—a rare and intense reaction to medication that causes severe skin damage and commonly affects the female genital tract. It happens in less than five people per one million per year.

† Oral, pill, patch, or IUD; tamoxifen; hormone replacement.

REASONS TO SUSPECT THAT HEAVY PERIODS ARE DUE TO A BROADER BLEEDING DISORDER

- Spontaneous nosebleeds within the past year
- Easily bruising (even without any immediate prior trauma)
- Minor wounds that bleed even though they are small
- Prolonged or heavy bleeding after dental procedures (e.g., tooth extraction, root canal)
- Unexpected bleeding after surgical procedures
- History of ovarian cyst hemorrhage
- Hemorrhage after childbirth, especially when the bleeding starts more than twenty-four hours after the birth
- Family history of bleeding disorder
- Heavy prolonged periods that do not improve with conventional treatments

Appendix C: Glossary and Gynecologic Subspecialty List*

Adenomyosis—When the endometrial tissue invades the myometrium, the muscle wall of the uterus. Happens concurrently with up to 30 percent of endometriosis cases.

Androgen—A "male" steroid sex hormone (e.g., testosterone) that occurs in all humans. Some drive male sex characteristics (e.g., testosterone), while others are precursors to estrogen. An essential component to many effective gynecologic treatments.

Anger squelching—The phenomenon too many Black women and femmes know all too well: "feeling the need to squelch or swallow strong feelings of anger." Has been found in research to be positively associated with fibroid risk over the lifetime.

Aromatase—An enzyme in the skin, fat cells, ovaries, and other places that converts androgens to estrogens. This is the reason you can make estrogen in places other than the ovary. The medications

* Italicized phrases are directly from *Merriam-Webster's Dictionary:* Merriam-Webster.com Dictionary, accessed April 21, 2025, https://www.merriam-webster.com/dictionary.

called *aromatase inhibitors* block this specific way of making estrogen in the body.

Atrophy—Broadly speaking, when tissue starts to thin out and weaken. Specifically, common in the endometrium and vulvar/vaginal tissues in the menopause phase of life.

Capillary—Very small blood vessels present throughout the body.

Carcinoma—A scientific word for the type of cancer that arises from glandular tissue in the body (as opposed to *stroma*). This is the most common type of endometrial cancer. There are several subtypes of carcinoma. From least to most aggressive: mucinous, endometrioid, serous, clear cell, and carcinosarcoma.

CBC (complete blood count)—A set of labs often measured together that gives information on red blood cells, white blood cells (markers of infection or inflammation), platelets (clotting cells), and other measures of your blood components.

Cycle syncing—A recently coined phrase that refers to organizing your daily activities (e.g., work, exercise, food) around the ovarian phases of the menstrual cycle. Most involve being active and visible during ovulatory phase and being restful and withdrawn during the late luteal phase. Some focus on specific types of exercise suitable for different phases. Biologically, there is no difference in metabolism, muscle building, or muscle breakdown over the different menstrual cycle phases. However, most people experience differences in energy levels, fatigue, pelvic discomfort or pain, cramping, and bloating during menstrual phases that would make some activities more or less appealing to do. In other words, it always makes sense to listen to your body and adjust your plans as you are able—whether you are cycling or not.

D&C (Dilation and curettage)—Dilation of the cervical os (opening) and curettage (removal of endometrial tissue with spoonlike instrument). Can be used to both diagnose and treat causes of abnormal and/or heavy menstrual bleeding. An outpatient surgical procedure.

Dysplasia—Abnormal changes to cells caused by mutations that often precede cancerous changes. In gynecology, most often refers to cervical, vaginal, or vulvar dysplasia.

Endometrial biopsy—A procedure to remove a sample of endometrial tissue to examine for causes of abnormal bleeding and/or infertility. Should always be done with adequate pain control measures as determined by the patient. Critical to perform if there is any concern for possible endometrial cancer, especially for Black women at risk.

Endometrial cancer—A cancer of the womb that grows from the inner lining of the uterus (the endometrium). One of the few cancers that is rising in number of cases each year. Will be more common than colon cancer by 2030. Black women have a higher chance of getting this cancer and more than double the risk of death.

Endometrial polyp—A growth of glandular tissue in the endometrium that can be benign (noncancerous) or cancerous. Can cause abnormal, irregular bleeding or spotting.

Endometriosis—The presence and growth of tissue similar to endometrium in places other than the uterus and especially in the pelvis and abdomen that often results in severe pain and infertility. An endometrioma is when endometriosis grows as a mass or cyst within an ovary. A condition that is underdiagnosed and underfunded because our society doesn't care about Womb Suffering.

Endometritis—Inflammation or infection of the endometrium, or inner lining of the womb.

Endometrium—The inner wall, or lining, of the uterus (womb) that has two layers—basal and superficial. During the menstrual cycle, the superficial layer grows and sheds in response to ovarian hormone signals.

Estrogen—Any of various natural steroids (e.g., estradiol) that are formed from androgen precursors, that are secreted chiefly by the ovaries, placenta, adipose tissue, and testes, and that stimulate the development of female secondary sex characteristics and promote the growth and maintenance of the female reproductive system. An essential component to many effective gynecologic treatments.

Ferritin—A measure of iron storage that is used to determine iron deficiency. Though the World Health Organization (and many labs) report levels under 15 are abnormal, most people have significant symptoms at levels below 26, and some symptoms below 50.

Heavy menstrual bleeding—Menstrual bleeding that is greater than 80 mL (2.7 fluid ounces) for a full cycle; menstrual bleeding that significantly negatively impacts quality of life; menstrual bleeding associated with a period longer than seven days, needing more than one heavy pad / tampon per hour for more than two hours, passing clots larger than one inch (quarter size); anemia due to menstrual bleeding. Usually takes three years before a woman is diagnosed, and less than a third of women ever get adequate treatment. A shame.

Hemoglobin/hematocrit—Both are labs used to measure your red blood cell count. The red blood cells, with the help of iron, deliver oxygen to all of your body and your brain. When the hemoglobin or hematocrit level is below normal, that is the clinical definition of being anemic.

Histology—The classification system for what human body tissues look like under the microscope. Different histology types—like in endometrial cancer—have different levels of mutations, aggressiveness, and therefore chance of survival when diagnosed.

Hormones—A product of living cells that circulates in body fluids (such as blood) and produces a specific, often stimulatory effect on the activity of cells usually remote from its point of origin. Often invoked in gynecology and/or women's health spaces to mean estrogen or progesterone derivatives. Also often used to dismiss dozens of effective and wildly different gynecologic therapies, as in "I don't want any hormones," or "You need to detox from hormones." See chapter 10 for the connection to misogyny.

Hysterectomy—Removal of the uterus (womb) via surgery. Can be abdominal (laparotomy), laparoscopic (through small incisions and using cameras), vaginal (through the vagina), or robotic (using small incisions and robotic cameras and equipment).

Complete/total/simple hysterectomy—removal of the uterus (womb), including the cervix. (Does not include removal of the fallopian tubes or ovaries.)

Partial/subtotal hysterectomy—removal of the uterus (womb) *without* the cervix. The uterus is cut just above the cervix and the cervix is left inside the body. (Does not include removal of the fallopian tubes or ovaries.)

IUD—Intrauterine device placed in the womb to treat endometrial hyperplasia and heavy menstrual bleeding, decrease endometriosis pain, manage irregular perimenopausal bleeding, and/or prevent pregnancy. Comes in different sizes and doses based on intended use and underlying diagnosis.

Leiomyoma—Fibroid. Smooth muscle noncancerous tumor that grows from uterine muscle cells. Rarely, can also grow outside of the uterus. Made up of muscle cells and extracellular matrix tissue.

Subserosal—Grows within the outer wall of the uterus. Can be pedunculated (hanging on a stalk). Can be quite large before pressure or bulk symptoms are noticed.

Intramural—Grows within the middle muscle layer of the uterine wall. Can cause excess pain with uterine cramping.

Submucosal—Grows just under the inner layer (endometrium) of the uterine wall. Often causes the most bleeding, even if small.

Leiomyosarcoma—Rare smooth muscle cancer that originates in mutated uterine muscle cancer cells. Requires removal of the uterus (complete hysterectomy) and often chemotherapy for treatment.

Menarche—The name for the first menstrual cycle in a person's life. Usually happens between nine and fourteen years old.

Menopause—The reproductive life phase where menstrual cycles have stopped due to an end to ovulation. This can occur due to surgery (ovarian removal), a disease, trauma, medication that causes premature ovarian failure, or the natural aging of the ovary. Menopause also tends to correspond to when a person has run out of all F's to give. Do not mess with these people.

Menorrhagia—A now-retired term that refers to abnormally heavy bleeding with menstrual cycles.

Menstruation—The phase in the menstrual cycle where the endometrium that has grown (hypertrophied) in preparation for a pregnancy sheds when no embryo implantation occurs, resulting in vaginal bleeding. If the hormonal signal to grow the endometrium is low or off (from medication or menopause), there is no menstruation. Also, all menstruation results in vaginal bleeding, but not all vaginal bleeding is from menstruation. (See appendix B, "83 Potential Causes of Abnormal Female Genital Bleeding.")

Secretory phase—The phase of the menstrual cycle where the endometrium begins to break down in response to an increase of progesterone signals from the ovary.

Proliferative phase—The phase of the menstrual cycle where the superficial layer of the endometrium is growing (proliferating) in response to estrogen stimulation from the ovary.

Luteal phase—The ovarian cycle phase that corresponds to the secretory endometrial phase.

Follicular phase—The ovarian cycle phase that corresponds to the proliferative endometrial phase.

Myomectomy—A surgery to remove fibroid(s) from within the uterus—or, less commonly, the ovary, fallopian tube, or broad ligament. Where the fibroid(s) is determines what surgical approach is used.

NSAIDs (non-steroidal anti-inflammatory drugs)—Keyword: *anti-inflammatory*. Excellent over-the-counter pain relief for menstrual cramps (driven by inflammatory phase of menstruation) and often part of multistep efforts to address other causes of pelvic pain. Part of the class of medications originally discovered in ancient times when willow bark (salicin) was used to relieve pain and inflammation. Salicin led to the creation of aspirin, and aspirin led to the synthesis of ibuprofen. Other NSAIDs include naproxen, indomethacin, and diclofenac.

Oophorectomy—Removal of the ovary.

Ovarian cystectomy—Removal of a cyst within the ovary. The ovary remains in the body.

Ovulation—A singular event where a mature follicle (egg) is released from the ovary in preparation for possible fertilization and pregnancy.

Pelvic inflammatory disease—Infection of any or all of the uterus, fallopian tubes, and ovaries, which may also involve the neighboring pelvic organs (e.g., bladder, colon). Most often caused by *chlamydia, gonorrhea,* or *mycoplasma genitalium.*

Pelvic MRI—A radiology study that uses magnetic fields and atomic physics to take detailed, still images of the pelvis and is often used in planning complex fibroid surgery. Very expensive ($$$$) and can be a fight to get covered with insurance companies.

Perimenopause—A lay, commonly used, and often vague term referring to the start of menopausal symptoms but prior to the end of all ovulation. Perimenopause could start as early as the thirties or as late as the fifties. There is no test for perimenopause, and many symptoms of perimenopause (i.e., weight gain, fatigue, loss of muscle mass) are also symptoms of aging. Keeping perimenopause vague and broad allows everything to be perimenopause and a lot of folks to make money. On the other hand, menopausal symptoms do commonly start years before the last period and can continue for years afterward. So, *perimenopause* is a functional term.

Peritoneum—The thin, somewhat elastic, deepest, and innermost lining of the body wall of the abdomen and pelvis. Often a site where endometriosis can implant and cause pain and other symptoms.

Progesterone—A steroid sex hormone that is secreted by the corpus luteum to prepare the endometrium for implantation and later by the placenta during pregnancy to prevent rejection of the developing embryo or fetus.

Progestin—A synthetic progesterone. An essential component to many effective gynecologic treatments.

Prostaglandins—*Unsaturated cyclic fatty acids* that act as hormone-like substances in many areas of the body, of relevance to the womb because they are chief players in the inflammatory cascade that is part of normal menstruation.

Salpingectomy—Removal of the fallopian tube.

Salpingo-oophorectomy—Removal of both tubes and ovaries.

Unilateral salpingo-oophorectomy (USO)—Removal of one fallopian tube and ovary.

Bilateral salpingo-oophorectomy (BSO)—Removal of both fallopian tubes and ovaries.

Somatic gene mutations—A mouthful. But an important concept to understand. Our genes are inherited from our biological parents, but their expression (impact) can be modified by mutations that happen during our lifetimes. These are called *somatic* mutations because we are not born with them. Some somatic mutations are random, and some are caused by environmental exposures to known toxins, chronic stress, and many other things we have yet to discover.

Stem cells—Cells in the body that are undifferentiated, meaning they retain the ability to transform into a specific type of tissue as needed for growth or repair.

TAH/BSO—A common abbreviation in medical records that means *total abdominal hysterectomy and bilateral salpingo-oophorectomy*. Removal of the uterus (with the cervix), both fallopian tubes, and both ovaries.

TLH/BSO—Same meaning except the hysterectomy was laparoscopic (done through small incisions).

TVUS (transvaginal ultrasound)—A procedure where an imaging device uses sound waves to take a picture of the pelvic organs. A TVUS includes a blunt vaginal probe that is inserted into the vagina to take close-up pictures of the cervix, endometrium, tubes, and ovaries. It creates the most accurate live image of the pelvis and can capture video as well.

Ureters—These are small, straw-like, hollow tubes that drain urine from the kidneys and empty it into the bladder. They are snuggled in the posterior body wall, very close to the ovaries and uterus in the pelvis. Because of this, serious gynecologic conditions like fibroids or endometriosis can block or inflame the ureters and cause kidney damage if untreated.

Uterine-sparing treatments—A somewhat lofty medical and research term used to describe all medical and surgical treatments for gynecologic conditions that do *not* require removal of the uterus. May be helpful vocabulary to use in a visit to be clear you want to discuss non-hysterectomy options.

Uterus—the female reproductive organ that has the capacity to safely grow a pregnancy; that can shed monthly or rest quietly for decades with equal health; that manifests diseases like endometriosis, adenomyosis, fibroids, and cancer; and that uniquely holds a spiritual, emotional, and physical space in many who are born with one.

Subserosa—The outer layer of the uterine wall.

Myometrium—The middle (muscle) layer of the uterine wall.

Endometrium—The inner wall, or lining, of the uterus (womb) that has two layers—basal and superficial.

Weathering—The public health and biological concept of how chronic stress from societal oppression causes the early aging and/or physiological dysfunction that results in increased frequency and/or severity of chronic disease in marginalized populations. In other words, why I needed to write this book.

TYPES OF GYNECOLOGY / GYNECOLOGISTS

General gynecologist—Completed four years of obstetrics and gynecology (OB-GYN) residency, which provides the longest and most comprehensive training in primary everyday gynecology. Training includes basic gynecologic surgery, outpatient medicine (puberty, contraception, gynecologic conditions, menopause), and hospital management of gynecologic emergencies.

Urogynecology and female pelvic medicine—Specialize in medical and surgical diagnosis and treatment of urinary incontinence, fecal incontinence, uterine and other pelvic organ prolapse. Includes treatment for postpartum pelvic trauma and dysfunction. After completing a four-year OB-GYN residency, they do an additional three years of surgical training in these areas. Female urologists also treat pelvic floor disorders but come from the background of urology (focus on male reproductive organs and treatment).

Reproductive endocrinology and infertility—Specialize in reproductive endocrine disorders and infertility diagnosis and treatment. Though they receive the most training in the hormonal physiology of PCOS and menopause, most practices are heavily focused on infertility alone. Hopefully this changes quickly. After completing a four-year OB-GYN residency, they do an additional three years of medical and procedural training to diagnose and treat infertility.

Gynecologic oncology—Specialize in medical and surgical treatment of ovarian, uterine, cervical, vulvar, and vaginal cancers using anti-cancer medications and complex surgery, including traditional and minimally invasive techniques. After completing the four-year OB-GYN residency, these doctors do an additional three to four years of medical and surgical training. The only oncology specialists who can do both the medical and surgical treatment for their patients, making it a uniquely holistic experience in cancer care. Because of the advanced surgical training, they also often do complex non-cancer gynecologic operations that may involve the bladder or bowel as well. My subspecialty and therefore the best one. Ahem.

Minimally invasive gynecologic surgeons (MIGS)—Specialize in doing (non-cancer-related) gynecologic surgeries through minimally invasive techniques of laparoscopy and robotic surgery. Often have practices focused on fibroids (myomectomy, hysterectomy, D&C), endometriosis, adenomyosis, and benign ovarian cysts. A surgically focused specialty, but many have deep experience with pelvic pain and medical management as well.

Complex family planning—Specialize in complex contraception, preconception counseling, and complex abortion services, in addition to general gynecology. Young folks! If you want someone to walk you through the hundreds of hormonal formulations possible to find your right match in terms of birth control, these are your people.

To my trans, nonbinary, and gender expansive people: Any and all of these gynecologic specialties can and should be gender affirming and welcoming places for basic reproductive organ care. The expertise of delivery of hormone therapy, puberty blockers, and other lifesaving treatments for you tend to reside with specific gynecologists, pediatric endocrinologists, and internal medicine and family medicine providers with a specialized focus. I hope this changes quickly, so anyone you go to can provide the care you deserve.

OTHER SPECIALISTS SPECIFICALLY TRAINED IN GYNECOLOGIC HEALTH

Family medicine physicians and nurse practitioners

Women's health nurse practitioners

Certified nurse midwives

References Cited, in Order of Appearance

Chapter 1

Doll KM, Puliaev R, Chor J, Roston A, Patel UA, Patel A. Detection of gynecologic cancers in indigent women in an urban inner-city hospital. *Int J Gynecol Cancer*. 2012;22(7):1113–1117. doi:10.1097/IGC.0b013e31825f7fa0.

Doll KM, Meng K, Basch EM, Gehrig PA, Brewster WR, Meyer AM. Gynecologic cancer outcomes in the elderly poor: A population-based study. *Cancer*. 2015;121(20):3591–3599. doi:10.1002/cncr.29541.

Winkler SS, Tian C, Casablanca Y, et al. Racial, ethnic and country of origin disparities in aggressive endometrial cancer histologic subtypes. *Gynecol Oncol*. 2024;184:31–42. doi:10.1016/j.ygyno.2024.01.009.

Bruegl AS, Joshi S, Batman S, Weisenberger M, Munro E, Becker T. Gynecologic cancer incidence and mortality among American Indian / Alaska Native women in the Pacific Northwest, 1996–2016. *Gynecol Oncol*. 2020;157(3):686–692. doi:10.1016/j.ygyno.2020.03.033.

Miller AK, Gordon JC, Curtis JW, Ajayakumar J, Schumacher FR, Avril S. The geographic context of racial disparities in aggressive endometrial cancer subtypes: integrating social and environmental aspects to discern biological outcomes. *Int J Environ Res Public Health*. 2022;19(14). Epub 20220715. doi:10.3390/ijerph19148613.

Schlumbrecht M, Wright K, George S. Unique considerations in early detection, risk, and awareness of endometrial cancer in black women. *Cancer Control*. 2023;30:10732748231202952. doi:10.1177/10732748231202952.

Temkin SM, Rimel BJ, Bruegl AS, Gunderson CC, Beavis AL, Doll KM. A contemporary framework of health equity applied to gynecologic cancer care: a Society of Gynecologic Oncology evidenced-based review. *Gynecol Oncol*. 2018;149(1):70–77. doi:10.1016/j.ygyno.2017.11.013.

Walker, Adria R. Beauty influencer Jessica Pettway died of cervical cancer following misdiagnosis. *The Guardian*. March 21, 2024. https://www.theguardian.com/us-news/2024/mar/21/jessica-pettway-death-cervical-cancer.

Bernardi LA, Ghant MS, Andrade C, Recht H, Marsh EE. The association between subjective assessment of menstrual bleeding and measures of iron deficiency anemia in premenopausal African-American women: a cross-sectional study. *BMC Women's Health*. 2016;16(1):50. Published August 15, 2016. doi:10.1186/s12905-016-0329-z.

Bougie O, Healey J, Singh SS. Behind the times: revisiting endometriosis and race. *Am J Obstet Gynecol*. 2019;221(1):35.e1–35.e5. doi:10.1016/j.ajog.2019.01.238.

Bougie O, Yap MI, Sikora L, Flaxman T, Singh S. Influence of race/ethnicity on prevalence and presentation of endometriosis: a systematic review and meta-analysis. *BJOG*. 2019;126(9):1104–1115. doi:10.1111/1471-0528.15692.

Robinson WR, Cheng MM, Howard AG, Carpenter WR, Brewster WR, Doll KM. For U.S. Black women, shift of hysterectomy to outpatient settings may have lagged behind White women: a claims-based analysis, 2011–2013. *BMC Health Serv Res*. 2017;17(1):526. Published August 4, 2017. doi:10.1186/s12913-017-2471-1.

Doll KM, Hempstead B, Alson J, Sage L, Lavallee DL. Assessment of pre-diagnostic experiences of Black women with endometrial cancer. *JAMA Network Open*. May 1, 2020;3(5):e204964. PMID: 32412636.

Chapter 2

Cooper Owens, D. The birth of American gynecology. In: *Medical Bondage: Race, Gender, and the Origins of American Gynecology*. Athens: University of Georgia Press, 2017:15–41.

Cooper Owens, D. Black women's experiences in slavery and medicine. In: *Medical Bondage: Race, Gender, and the Origins of American Gynecology*. Athens: University of Georgia Press, 2017:47–56.

Kapsalis, Terri. *Public Privates: Performing Gynecology from Both Ends of the Speculum*. Durham, NC: Duke University Press, 1997:46. Archived from the original on December 17, 2019. Retrieved September 1, 2017, via Google Books.

Christmas, M. #SayHerName: should obstetrics and gynecology reckon with the legacy of JM Sims? *Reprod Sci*. 2021;28(11): 3282–3284. doi:10.1007/s43032-021-00567-6.

Anarcha, Lucy, and Betsey: the mothers of gynecology. https://www.anarchalucybetsey.org/.

Vernon LF. J. Marion Sims, MD: why he and his accomplishments need to continue to be recognized a commentary and historical review. *J Natl Med Assoc*. 2019;111(4):436–446. doi:10.1016/j.jnma.2019.02.002.

Hoffman KM, Trawalter S, Axt JR, Oliver MN. Racial bias in pain assessment and treatment recommendations, and false beliefs about biological differences between blacks and whites. *Proc Natl Acad Sci USA*. 2016;113(16):4296–4301. doi:10.1073/pnas.1516047113.

Johnson JD, Asiodu IV, McKenzie CP, et al. Racial and ethnic inequities in postpartum pain evaluation and management. *Obstet Gynecol*. 2019;134(6):1155–1162. doi:10.1097/AOG.0000000000003505.

Check DK, Samuel CA, Rosenstein DL, Dusetzina SB. Investigation of racial disparities in early supportive medication use and end-of-life care among Medicare beneficiaries with stage IV breast cancer. *J Clin Oncol*. 2016;34(19):2265–2270. doi:10.1200/JCO.2015.64.8162.

Allen JM, Awunti M, Guo Y, et al. Unraveling racial disparities in supportive care medication use among end-of-life pancreatic cancer patients: focus on pain management and psychiatric therapies. *Cancer Epidemiol Biomarkers Prev*. 2023;32(12):1675–1682. doi:10.1158/1055-9965.EPI-23-0251.

Check DK, Reeder-Hayes KE, Basch EM, Zullig LL, Weinberger M, Dusetzina SB. Investigating racial disparities in use of NK1 receptor antagonists to prevent chemotherapy-induced nausea and vomiting among women with breast cancer. *Breast Cancer Res Treat.* 2016;156(2):351–359. doi:10.1007/s10549-016-3747-6.

Woods Giscombé CL. Superwoman schema: African American women's views on stress, strength, and health. *Qual Health Res.* 2010;20(5):668–683. doi:10.1177/1049732310361892.

Cousin L. Cardio-oncology disparities: interplay of psychosocial stress, inflammation, and cardiometabolic health among Black breast cancer survivors. *Am Heart J Plus.* 2024;38:100366. Published January 30, 2024. doi:10.1016/j.ahjo.2024.100366.

Erving CL, Zajdel RA, Blevins KM, et al. The association between Superwoman schema and subjective sleep quality among Black women. *Sleep Health.* 2024;10(3):302–307. doi:10.1016/j.sleh.2023.12.008.

Thomas MD, Mendez RM, Zhang Y, et al. Superwoman schema, racial identity, and cellular aging among African American women. *Gerontologist.* 2022;62(5):762–772. doi:10.1093/geront/gnac005.

Perez AD, Dufault SM, Spears EC, Chae DH, Woods Giscombé CL, Allen AM. Superwoman schema and John Henryism among African American women: an intersectional perspective on coping with racism. *Soc Sci Med.* 2023;316:115070. doi:10.1016/j.socscimed.2022.115070.

Stevens KR, Masters KS, Imoukhuede PI, et al. Fund Black scientists. *Cell.* 2021;184(3):561–565. doi:10.1016/j.cell.2021.01.011.

Hoppe TA, Litovitz A, Willis KA, et al. Topic choice contributes to the lower rate of NIH awards to African-American/black scientists. *Sci Adv.* 2019;5(10):eaaw7238. Published October 9, 2019. doi:10.1126/sciadv.aaw7238.

National Academies of Sciences, Engineering, and Medicine. *A New Vision for Women's Health Research: Transformative Change at the National Institutes of Health.* Washington, DC: National Academies Press, 2025. https://doi.org/10.17226/28586.

Office of Research on Women's Health. *Perspectives on Advancing NIH Research on the Health of Women.* Washington, DC: National Institutes of Health, 2023. Accessed May 2, 2025. https://orwh.od.nih.gov/sites/orwh/files/docs/ORWH_WHC_ExecutiveSummary508.pdf.

Skloot, Rebecca. *The Immortal Life of Henrietta Lacks*. New York: Crown, 2010.

"The Legacy of Henrietta Lacks." Johns Hopkins Medicine. https://www.hopkinsmedicine.org/henrietta-lacks.

Doll KM. Minority enrollment on clinical trials enhances scientific rigor but requires structural changes and commitment. *Gynecologic Oncology*. 2020;157(2):301–302. PMID: 3238919.

Chapter 3 (used throughout chapter)

Jain V, Chodankar RR, Maybin JA, Critchley HOD. Uterine bleeding: how understanding endometrial physiology underpins menstrual health. *Nat Rev Endocrinol.* 2022;18(5):290–308. doi:10.1038/s41574-021-00629-4.

Critchley HOD, Maybin JA, Armstrong GM, Williams ARW. Physiology of the endometrium and regulation of menstruation. *Physiol Rev*. 2020;100(3):1149–1179. doi:10.1152/physrev.00031.2019.

Critchley HOD, Babayev E, Bulun SE, et al. Menstruation: science and society. *Am J Obstet Gynecol*. 2020;223(5):624–664. doi:10.1016/j.ajog.2020.06.004.

Wright MA, Doll KM, Myers E, Carpenter WR, Gartner DR, Robinson WR. Changing trends in Black-White racial differences in surgical menopause: a population-based study. *Am J Obstet Gynecol*. 2021;225(5):502.e1–502.e13. doi:10.1016/j.ajog.2021.05.045.

Lacroix AE, Gondal H, Shumway KR, Langaker MD. Physiology, menarche. In: *StatPearls*. Treasure Island, FL: StatPearls Publishing, March 11, 2023.

Chapter 4

Bernardi LA, Ghant MS, Andrade C, Recht H, Marsh EE. The association between subjective assessment of menstrual bleeding and measures of iron deficiency anemia in premenopausal African-American women: a cross-sectional study. *BMC Women's Health*. 2016;16(1):50. Published August 15, 2016. doi:10.1186/s12905-016-0329-z.

da Silva Filho AL, Caetano C, Lahav A, Grandi G, Lamaita RM. The difficult journey to treatment for women suffering from heavy menstrual bleeding: a multi-national survey. *Eur J Contracept Reprod Health Care*. 2021;26(5):390–398. doi:10.1080/13625187.2021.1925881.

Munro MG, Mast AE, Powers JM, et al. The relationship between heavy menstrual bleeding, iron deficiency, and iron deficiency anemia. *Am J Obstet Gynecol.* 2023;229(1):1–9. doi:10.1016/j.ajog.2023.01.017.

Harvey SV, Pfeiffer RM, Landy R, Wentzensen N, Clarke MA. Trends and predictors of hysterectomy prevalence among women in the United States. *Am J Obstet Gynecol.* 2022; 227(4):611.e1–611.e12. doi:10.1016/j.ajog.2022.06.028.

Doll KM, Dusetzina SB, Robinson W. Trends in inpatient and outpatient hysterectomy and oophorectomy rates among commercially insured women in the United States, 2000–2014. *JAMA Surg.* 2016; 151(9):876–877. doi:10.1001/jamasurg.2016.0804.

Robinson WR, Cheng MM, Howard AG, Carpenter WR, Brewster WR, Doll KM. For U.S. Black women, shift of hysterectomy to outpatient settings may have lagged behind White women: a claims-based analysis, 2011–2013. *BMC Health Serv Res.* 2017; 17(1):526. Published August 4, 2017. doi:10.1186/s12913-017-2471-1.

Doll KM, Howard AG, Stürmer T, et al. Development of an algorithm to assess unmeasured symptom severity in gynecologic care. *Am J Obstet Gynecol.* 2022; 226(3):388.e1–388.e11. doi:10.1016/j.ajog.2021.11.020.

Robinson WR, Mathias JG, Wood ME, et al. Ethnoracial differences in premenopausal hysterectomy: the role of symptom severity. *Obstet Gynecol.* 2023;142(2):350–359 PMID: 37473411.

Salcedo AC, Yun J, Carter C, Hart E. Therapeutic carbohydrate restriction as a metabolic modality for the prevention and treatment of abnormal uterine bleeding. *Nutrients.* 2023;15(17):3760. Published August 28, 2023. doi:10.3390/nu15173760.

Jewson M, Purohit P, Lumsden MA. Progesterone and abnormal uterine bleeding/menstrual disorders. *Best Pract Res Clin Obstet Gynaecol.* 2020;69:62–73. doi:10.1016/j.bpobgyn.2020.05.004.

Douglas N, Lobo RA. Reproductive endocrinology. In: *Comprehensive Gynecology*, 8th ed. Philadelphia: Elsevier, 2022:76–105.

Chapter 5

Bougie O, Healey J, Singh SS. Behind the times: revisiting endometriosis and race. *Am J Obstet Gynecol.* 2019;221(1):35.e1–35.e5. doi:10.1016/j.ajog.2019.01.238.

Zondervan KT, Becker CM, Missmer SA. Endometriosis. *N Engl J Med*. 2020;382(13):1244–1256. doi:10.1056/NEJMra1810764.

As-Sanie S, Mackenzie SC, Morrison L, et al. Endometriosis: a review. *JAMA*. 2025;334(1):64–78. doi:10.1001/jama.2025.2975.

Carey ET, Wong JMK, Khan Z. Comprehensive review of endometriosis care. *Obstet Gynecol*. 2025;146(3):323–340. Published July 17, 2025. doi:10.1097/AOG.0000000000006004.

Shafrir AL, Farland LV, Shah DK, et al. Risk for and consequences of endometriosis: a critical epidemiologic review. *Best Pract Res Clin Obstet Gynaecol*. 2018;51:1–15. doi:10.1016/j.bpobgyn.2018.06.001.

Katon JG, Plowden TC, Marsh EE. Racial disparities in uterine fibroids and endometriosis: a systematic review and application of social, structural, and political context. *Fertil Steril*. 2023;119(3):355–363. doi:10.1016/j.fertnstert.2023.01.022.

Shigesi N, Harris HR, Fang H, et al. The phenotypic and genetic association between endometriosis and immunological diseases. *Hum Reprod*. Published online April 22, 2025. doi:10.1093/humanrep/deaf062.

Bleil ME, Appelhans BM, Gregorich SE, Hiatt RA, Roisman GI, Booth-LaForce C. Pubertal timing: a life course pathway linking early life risk to adulthood cardiometabolic health. *PLOS One*. 2024;19(3):e0299433. Published March 27, 2024. doi:10.1371/journal.pone.0299433.

Chumlea WC, Schubert CM, Roche AF, et al. Age at menarche and racial comparisons in US girls. *Pediatrics*. 2003;111(1):110–113. doi:10.1542/peds.111.1.110.

Brichant G, Laraki I, Henry L, Munaut C, Nisolle M. New therapeutics in endometriosis: a review of hormonal, non-hormonal, and non-coding RNA treatments. *Int J Mol Sci*. 2021;22(19):10498. Published September 28, 2021. doi:10.3390/ijms221910498.

https://www.nice.org.uk/guidance/ta1057/evidence/final-draft-guidance-committee-papers-pdf-15304905902. Single technology appraisal: relugolix-estradiol-norethisterone acetate for treating symptoms of endometriosis. 2025. ID3982. National Institute for Health and Care Excellence. Accessed May 9, 2025.

Bower JK, Schreiner PJ, Sternfeld B, Lewis CE. Black-White differences in hysterectomy prevalence: the CARDIA study. *Am J Public Health*. 2009;99(2):300–307. doi:10.2105/AJPH.2008.133702.

Robinson WR, Cheng MM, Howard AG, Carpenter WR, Brewster WR, Doll KM. For U.S. Black women, shift of hysterectomy to outpatient settings may have lagged behind White women: a claims-based analysis, 2011–2013. *BMC Health Serv Res*. 2017; 17(1):526. Published August 4, 2017. doi:10.1186/s12913-017-2471-1.

Robinson WR, Mathias JG, Wood ME, et al. Ethnoracial differences in premenopausal hysterectomy: the role of symptom severity. *Obstet Gynecol*. 2023;142(2):350–359. doi:10.1097/AOG.0000000000005225.

Doll KM, Howard AG, Stürmer T, et al. Development of an algorithm to assess unmeasured symptom severity in gynecologic care. *Am J Obstet Gynecol*. 2022;226(3):388.e1–388.e11. doi:10.1016/j.ajog.2021.11.020.

Penn M, Colley D, Koirala P, King L, Fitzgerald J. Price and prejudice: reimbursement of surgical care on male versus female anatomies. *J Women's Health (Larchmt)*. February 21, 2025. doi:10.1089/jwh.2024.0984. Epub ahead of print. PMID: 39978776.

Nirgianakis K, Egger K, Kalaitzopoulos DR, Lanz S, Bally L, Mueller MD. Effectiveness of dietary interventions in the treatment of endometriosis: a systematic review. *Reprod Sci.* 2022;29(1):26–42. doi: 10.1007/s43032-020-00418-w.

Zheng SH, Chen XX, Chen Y, et al. Antioxidant vitamins supplementation reduce endometriosis related pelvic pain in humans: a systematic review and meta-analysis. *Reprod Biol Endocrinol* 21. Article number 79 (2023). https://doi.org/10.1186/s12958-023-01126-1.

Bayu P, Wibisono JJ. Vitamin C and E antioxidant supplementation may significantly reduce pain symptoms in endometriosis: a systematic review and meta-analysis of randomized controlled trials. *PLOS One*. 2024;19(5):e0301867. Published May 31, 2024. doi:10.1371/journal.pone.0301867.

Li Y, Hung S-W, Zhang R, et al. Melatonin in endometriosis: mechanistic understanding and clinical insight. *Nutrients*. 2022;14(19):4087. https://doi.org/10.3390/nu14194087.

Schwertner A, Conceição Dos Santos CC, Costa GD, et al. Efficacy of melatonin in the treatment of endometriosis: a phase II, randomized, double-blind, placebo-controlled trial. *Pain*. 2013;154(6):874–881. doi:10.1016/j.pain.2013.02.025.

Koller D, Pathak GA, Wendt FR, et al. Epidemiologic and genetic associations of endometriosis with depression, anxiety, and eating disorders. *JAMA Netw Open*. 2023;6(1):e2251214. doi:10.1001/jamanetworkopen.2022.51214.

Davis A. The legacy of slavery: standard for a new womanhood. In: *Women, Race & Class*. New York: Vintage, 1983:7–28.

Schulman KA, Berlin JA, Harless W, et al. The effect of race and sex on physicians' recommendations for cardiac catheterization [published correction appears in *N Engl J Med*. 1999;340(14):1130]. *N Engl J Med*. 1999;340(8);618–626. doi:/10/1056/NEJM199902253400806.

Cromeens MG, Thoyre S, Carey ET, Knafl K, Robinson WR. Inquiry into women's pathways to diagnosis of endometriosis: a qualitative study protocol. *J Adv Nurs*. 2021;77(2):1017–1026. doi:10.1111/jan.14616.

Culley L, Law C, Hudson N, et al. The social and psychological impact of endometriosis on women's lives: a critical narrative review. *Hum Reprod Update*. 2013;19(6):625–639.

Denny, E. "You are one of the unlucky ones": delay in the diagnosis of endometriosis. *Divers Health Social Care*. 2004;1(1):39–44.

Soliman AM, Fuldeore M, Snabes MC. Factors associated with time to endometriosis diagnosis in the United States. *J Women's Health (Larchmt)*. 2017;26(7):788–797. doi:10.1089/jwh.2016.6003.

Young K, Fisher J, Kirkman M. Women's experiences of endometriosis: a systematic review and synthesis of qualitative research. *J Fam Plann Reprod Health Care*. 2015;41(3):225–234.

Chapter 6

Upadhyay S, Dubey PK. Gene variants polymorphisms and uterine leiomyoma: an updated review. *Front Genet.* 2024;15:1330807. doi:10.3389/fgene.2024.1330807.

Marsh EE, Ekpo GE, Cardozo ER, Brocks M, Dune T, Cohen LS. Racial differences in fibroid prevalence and ultrasound findings in asymptomatic young women (18–30 years old): a pilot study. *Fertil Steril*. 2013;99(7):1951–1957. doi:10.1016/j.fertnstert.2013.02.017. Epub March 15, 2013. PMID: 23498888; PMCID: PMC4465811.

Giuliani E, As-Sanie S, Marsh EE. Epidemiology and management of uterine fibroids. *Int J Gynaecol Obstet*. 2020;149(1):3–9. doi:10.1002/ijgo.13102. Epub February 17, 2020. PMID: 31960950.

Baird DD, Dunson DB, Hill MC, Cousins D, Schectman JM. High cumulative incidence of uterine leiomyoma in black and white women: ultrasound evidence. *Am J Obstet Gynecol* 2003;188: 100–110.

Bulun SE. Uterine fibroids. *N Engl J Med.* 2013;369(14):1344–1355. doi:10.1056/NEJMra1209993. PMID: 24088094.

Wise LA, Palmer JR, Harlow BL, et al. Reproductive factors, hormonal contraception, and risk of uterine leiomyomata in African-American women: a prospective study. *Am J Epidemiol.* 2004;159(2):113–123. doi:10.1093/aje/kwh016.

Wise LA, Palmer JR, Spiegelman D, et al. Influence of body size and body fat distribution on risk of uterine leiomyomata in U.S. black women. *Epidemiology.* 2005;16(3):346–354. doi:10.1097/01.ede.0000158742.11877.99.

Baird DD, Dunson DB, Hill MC, Cousins D, Schectman JM. Association of physical activity with development of uterine leiomyoma. *Am J Epidemiol.* 2007;165(2):157–163. doi:10.1093/aje/kwj363.

Wise LA, Radin RG, Palmer JR, Kumanyika SK, Rosenberg L. A prospective study of dairy intake and risk of uterine leiomyomata. *Am J Epidemiol.* 2010;171(2):221–232. doi:10.1093/aje/kwp355.

Brasky TM, Bethea TN, Wesselink AK, Wegienka GR, Baird DD, Wise LA. Dietary fat intake and risk of uterine leiomyomata: a prospective ultrasound study. *Am J Epidemiol.* 2020;189(12): 1538–1546. doi:10.1093/aje/kwaa097.

Wise LA, Palmer JR, Harlow BL, et al. Risk of uterine leiomyomata in relation to tobacco, alcohol and caffeine consumption in the Black Women's Health Study. *Hum Reprod.* 2004;19(8):1746–1754. doi:10.1093/humrep/deh30.

Wise LA, Laughlin-Tommaso SK. Epidemiology of uterine fibroids: from menarche to menopause. *Clin Obstet Gynecol.* 2016;59(1):2–24. doi:10.1097/GRF.0000000000000164.

Palmer JR, Cozier YC, Rosenberg L. Research on health disparities: strategies and findings from the Black Women's Health Study. *Am J Epidemiol.* 2023;192(11):1806–1810. doi:10.1093/aje/kwac022. PMID: 35136921; PMCID: PMC11004793.

Radin RG, Palmer JR, Rosenberg L, Kumanyika SK, Wise LA. Dietary glycemic index and load in relation to risk of uterine leiomyomata in the Black Women's Health Study. *Am J Clin Nutr.* 2010;91(5):1281–1288. doi:10.3945/ajcn.2009.28698.

Langton CR, Harmon QE, Upson K, Baird DD. Soy-based infant formula feeding and uterine fibroid development in a prospective ultrasound study of Black/African-American women. *Environ Health Perspect*. 2023;131(1):17006. doi:10.1289/EHP11089.

Krzyżanowski J, Paszkowski T, Woźniak S. The role of nutrition in pathogenesis of uterine fibroids. *Nutrients*. 2023;15(23):4984. Published December 1, 2023. doi:10.3390/nu15234984.

Xu F, Li F, Li L, Lin D, Hu H, Shi Q. Vitamin D as a risk factor for the presence of asymptomatic uterine fibroids in premenopausal Han Chinese women. *Fertil Steril*. 2021;115(5):1288–1293. doi:10.1016/j.fertnstert.2020.12.001.

Combs A, Singh B, Nylander E, et al. A systematic review of vitamin D and fibroids: pathophysiology, prevention, and treatment. *Reprod Sci.* 2023;30:1049–1064. doi.org/10.1007/s43032-022-01011-z.

Harmon QE, Patchel SA, Denslow S, et al. Vitamin D and uterine fibroid growth, incidence, and loss: a prospective ultrasound study. *Fertil Steril.* 2022;118(6):1127–1136. doi:10.1016/j.fertnstert.2022.08.851.

Sabry M, Halder SK, Ait Allah AS, Roshdy E, Rajaratnam V, Al-Hendy A. Serum vitamin D3 level inversely correlates with uterine fibroid volume in different ethnic groups: a cross-sectional observational study. *Int J Women's Health*. 2013;5:93–100.

Baird DD, Hill MC, Schectman JM, Hollis BW. Vitamin D and the risk of uterine fibroids. *Epidemiology*. 2013;24(3):447–453. doi:10.1097/EDE.0b013e31828acca0.

Paffoni A, Somigliana E, Vigano P, et al. Vitamin D status in women with uterine leiomyomas. *J Clin Endocrinol Metab.* 2013;98(8):E1374–E1378.

Vines AI, Nguyen TTX, Ta M, Esserman D, Baird DD. Self-reported daily stress, squelching of anger and the management of daily stress and the prevalence of uterine leiomyomata: the ultrasound screening study. *Stress Health*. 2011;27:e188–e194.

Boynton-Jarrett R, Rich-Edwards JW, Jun HJ, Hibert EN, Wright RJ. Abuse in childhood and risk of uterine leiomyoma: the role of emotional support in biologic resilience. *Epidemiology*. 2011;22(1):6–14. doi:10.1097/EDE.0b013e3181ffb172. PMID: 21068667; PMCID: PMC4010091.

Wise LA, Palmer JR, Reich D, Cozier YC, Rosenberg L. Hair relaxer use and risk of uterine leiomyomata in African-American women.

Am J Epidemiol. 2012;175(5):432–440. doi:10.1093/aje/kwr351. Epub January 10, 2012. PMID: 22234483; PMCID: PMC3282879.

Liu J, Clark LP, Bechle MJ, et al. Disparities in air pollution exposure in the United States by race/ethnicity and income, 1990–2010. *Environ Health Perspect*. 2021;129(12):127005. doi:10.1289/EHP8584. Epub December 15, 2021. PMID: 34908495; PMCID: PMC8672803.

Rumph JT, Stephens VR, Martin JL, et al. Uncovering evidence: associations between environmental contaminants and disparities in women's health. *Int J Environ Res Public Health*. 2022;19:1257. https://doi.org/10.3390/ijerph19031257.

Huyck KL, Panhuysen CI, Cuenco KT, et al. The impact of race as a risk factor for symptom severity and age at diagnosis of uterine leiomyomata among affected sisters. *Am J Obstet Gynecol*. 2008;198(2):168.e1–168.e9. doi:10.1016/j.ajog.2007.05.038. PMID: 18226615; PMCID: PMC2265083.

Baird DD, Dunson DB, Hill MC, Cousins D, Schectman JM. High cumulative incidence of uterine leiomyoma in black and white women: ultrasound evidence. *Am J Obstet Gynecol*. 2003;188:100–107.

Peddada SD, Laughlin SK, Miner K, et al. Growth of uterine leiomyomata among premenopausal black and white women. *Proc Natl Acad Sci USA*. 2008;105(50):19887–19892. doi:10.1073/pnas.0808188105. Epub December 1, 2008. PMID: 19047643; PMCID: PMC2604959.

Anchan RM, Spies JB, Zhang S, et al. Long-term health-related quality of life and symptom severity following hysterectomy, myomectomy, or uterine artery embolization for the treatment of symptomatic uterine fibroids. *Am J Obstet Gynecol*. 2023;229:275.e1–275.e17.

Ghant MS, Sengoba KS, Recht H, Cameron KA, Lawson AK, Marsh EE. Beyond the physical: a qualitative assessment of the burden of symptomatic uterine fibroids on women's emotional and psychosocial health. *J Psychosom Res*. 2015;78(5):499–503. doi:10.1016/j.jpsychores.2014.12.016. Epub February 2, 2015. PMID: 25725565.

Stewart EA, Nicholson WK, Bradley L, Borah BJ. The burden of uterine fibroids for African-American women: results of a national survey. *J Womens Health (Larchmt)*. 2013;22:807–816.

Combs A, Singh B, Nylander E, et al. A systematic review of vitamin D and fibroids: pathophysiology, prevention, and treatment. *Reprod Sci.* 2023;30(4):1049–1064. doi:10.1007/s43032-022-01011-z. Epub August 12, 2022. PMID: 35960442.

Parsanezhad ME, Azmoon M, Alborzi S, et al. A randomized, controlled clinical trial comparing the effects of aromatase inhibitor (letrozole) and gonadotropin-releasing hormone agonist (triptorelin) on uterine leiomyoma volume and hormonal status. *Fertil Steril.* 2010;93(1):192–198. doi:10.1016/j.fertnstert.2008.09.064.

Arnreiter C, Oppelt P. A systematic review of the treatment of uterine myomas using transcervical ultrasound-guided radiofrequency ablation with the SONATA system. *J Minim Invasive Gynecol.* 2021;28(8):1462–1469. doi:10.1016/j.jmig.2021.04.009.

Chudnoff SG et al. Outpatient procedure for the treatment and relief of symptomatic uterine myomas. *Obstet Gynecol.* 2013;121(5):1075–1082.

Miller CE, Osman KM. Transcervical radiofrequency ablation of symptomatic uterine fibroids: 2-year results of the SONATA pivotal trial. *J Gynecol Surg.* 2019;35(6):345–349.

Baird DD, Patchel SA, Saldana TM, et al. Uterine fibroid incidence and growth in an ultrasound-based, prospective study of young African Americans. *Am J Obstet Gynecol.* 2020;223(3):402.e1–402.e18. doi:10.1016/j.ajog.2020.02.016. Epub February 24, 2020. PMID: 32105679; PMCID: PMC8039858.

Peddada SD, Laughlin SK, Miner K, et al. Growth of uterine leiomyomata among premenopausal black and white women. *Proc Natl Acad Sci USA.* 2008;105(50):19887–19892. doi:10.1073/pnas.0808188105. Epub December 1, 2008. PMID: 19047643; PMCID: PMC2604959.

Chapter 7

Lu KH, Broaddus RR. Endometrial cancer. *N Engl J Med.* 2020;383(21):2053–2064. doi:10.1056/NEJMra1514010.

Siegel RL, Giaquinto AN, Jemal A. Cancer statistics, 2024. *CA Cancer J Clin.* 2024;74(1):12–49. doi:10.3322/caac.21820.

Rahib L, Smith BD, Aizenberg R, et al. Projecting cancer incidence and deaths to 2030: the unexpected burden of thyroid, liver, and pancreas cancers in the United States. *Cancer Res.* 2014;74(11):2913–2921. doi: 0.1158/0008-5472.CAN-14-0155.

Gaber C, Meza R, Ruterbusch JJ, Cote ML. Endometrial cancer trends by race and histology in the USA: projecting the number of new cases from 2015 to 2040. *J Racial Ethn Health Disparities*. Published online October 17, 2016. doi:10.1007/s40615-016-0292-2.

"SEER*Explorer: An Interactive Website for SEER Cancer Statistics 2023." Cancer Surveillance Research Program—National Cancer Institute. Accessed May 21, 2025. https://seer.cancer.gov/statistics-network/explorer/application.html.

Doll KM, Winn AN, Goff BA. Untangling the Black-White mortality gap in endometrial cancer: a cohort simulation. *AJOG*. 2017;216(3):324–325. PMID: 2803465.

Doll KM, Winn A, Goff BA. Assessing endometrial cancer risk among US women: long-term trends using hysterectomy-adjusted analysis. *AJOG*. 2019;221(4):318.e1–318.e9. PMID: 31125544.

Saka AH, Giaquinto AN, McCullough LE, et al. Cancer statistics for African American and Black people, 2025. *CA Cancer J Clin*. 2025;75(2):111–140. doi:10.3322/caac.21874.

Winkler SS, Tian C, Casablanca Y, et al. Racial, ethnic and country of origin disparities in aggressive endometrial cancer histologic subtypes. *Gynecol Oncol*. 2024;184:31–42. doi:10.1016/j.ygyno.2024.01.009.

Clarke MA, Devesa SS, Hammer A, Wentzensen N. Racial and ethnic differences in hysterectomy-corrected uterine corpus cancer mortality by stage and histologic subtype. *JAMA Oncol*. 2022;8(6):895–903. doi:10.1001/jamaoncol.2022.0009.

Paramsothy P, Harlow SD, Greendale GA, et al. Bleeding patterns during the menopausal transition in the multi-ethnic Study of Women's Health Across the Nation (SWAN): a prospective cohort study. *BJOG*. 2014;121(12):1564–1573. doi:10.1111/1471–0528.12768.

Ford CL, Airhihenbuwa CO. The public health critical race methodology: praxis for antiracism research. *Soc Sci Med.* 2010;71(8):1390–1398. doi: 0.1016/j.socscimed.2010.07.030.

Doll KM. Investigating Black-White disparities in gynecologic oncology: theories, conceptual models, and applications. *Gynecol Oncol*. 2018;149(1):78–83. PMID: 29605054.

Doll KM, Snyder CR, Ford CL. Endometrial cancer disparities: a race-conscious critique of the literature. *AJOG*. 2018;218(5):474–482.e2. PMID: 28964822.

Doll KM. Endometrial cancer and reproductive justice. *Obstet Gynecol.* 2023;142(3):477–480. PMID: 37590979.

Doll KM, Khor S, Odem-Davis K, et al. Role of bleeding recognition and evaluation in Black-White disparities in endometrial cancer. *AJOG*. 2018;219(6):593.e1–593.e14. PMID: 30291839.

ACOG committee opinion no. 734: the role of transvaginal ultrasonography in evaluating the endometrium of women with postmenopausal bleeding. *Obstet Gynecol.* 2018;131(5):e124–e129. doi:10.1097/AOG.0000000000002631. Original opinion No. 440, published in 2008, no longer available.

Doll KM, Hempstead B, Alson J, Sage L, Lavallee DL. Assessment of pre-diagnostic experiences of Black women with endometrial cancer. *JAMA Netw Open.* 2020;3(5):e204964. PMID: 32412636.

Doll KM, Romano SS, Marsh EE, Robinson WR. Estimated performance of transvaginal ultrasonography for evaluation of postmenopausal bleeding in a simulated cohort of Black and White women in the US. *JAMA Oncol.* 2021;7(8):1158–1165. PMID: 34264304.

Romano S, Doll KM. The impact of fibroids and histologic subtype on the performance of U.S. clinical guidelines for the diagnosis of endometrial cancer among Black women. *Ethn Dis.* 2020;30(4):543–552. eCollection 2020 Fall. PMID: 32989354.

Doll KM, Nguyen A, Alson JA. A conceptual model of vulnerability to care delay among women at risk for endometrial cancer. *Gynecol Oncol.* 2022;164(2):318–324. PMID: 34862064.

Reeves A, Elliott MR, Karvonen-Gutierrez CA, Harlow SD. Systematic exclusion at study commencement masks earlier menopause for Black women in the Study of Women's Health Across the Nation (SWAN). *Int J Epidemiol.* 2023;52(5):1612–1623. doi:10.1093/ije/dyad085.

Harlow SD, Burnett-Bowie SM, Greendale GA, et al. Disparities in reproductive aging and midlife health between black and white women: the Study of Women's Health Across the Nation (SWAN) [published correction appears in *Women's Midlife Health.* 2022;8(1):10. doi:10.1186/s40695-022-00082-x]. *Women's Midlife Health.* 2022;8(1):3. Published February 8, 2022. doi:10.1186/s40695-022-00073-y.

Sage L, Dwyer E, Gray DA, et al. Endometrial cancer knowledge and guideline concordant practice patterns among first-line providers.

J Womens Health. August 1, 2023. Epub ahead of print. PMID: 37527205.

Rios-Doria E, Parker EU, Kohrn BF, et al. TP53 somatic evolution in the normal endometrium of Black and White individuals. *Gynecol Oncol*. Published online April 17, 2025. doi:10.1016/j.ygyno.2025.04.002.

Bruegl AS, Joshi S, Batman S, Weisenberger M, Munro E, Becker T. Gynecologic cancer incidence and mortality among American Indian / Alaska Native women in the Pacific Northwest, 1996–2016. *Gynecol Oncol*. 2020;157(3):686–692. doi:10.1016/j.ygyno.2020.03.033.

Doll KM, Suri A, Gehrig PA. Minimally invasive surgery in endometrial cancer: recent updates. *Expert Rev Obstet Gynecol*. 2013:8(3):271–283. doi:10.1586/eog.13.14.

Rowinsky EK, Donehower RC. Paclitaxel (taxol) [published correction appears in *N Engl J Med*. 1995;333(1):75]. *N Engl J Med*. 1995;332(15):1004–1014. doi:10.1056/NEJM199504133321507.

Hamilton CA, Pothuri B, Arend RC, et al. Endometrial cancer: a society of gynecologic oncology evidence-based review and recommendations. *Gynecol Oncol*. 2021;160(3):817–826. doi:10.1016/j.ygyno.2020.12.021.

Orlando MS, Bradley LD. Implementation of office hysteroscopy for the evaluation and treatment of intrauterine pathology. *Obstet Gynecol*. 2022;140(3):499–513. doi:10.1097/AOG.0000000000004898.

Doll KM, Hempstead B, Truitt AR. Seeking Black women's voices in endometrial cancer research via deliberate community engagement. *Progr Community Health Partnersh*. 2019;13(3):253–264. PMID: 31564666.

Alson JA, Nguyen A, Hempstead B, et al. "We are a powerful movement": evaluation of an endometrial cancer education program for Black women. *Progress Community Health Partnersh*. 2021;15(4):439–452. PMID: 34975026.

Gamble CR, Sage L, Nguyen A, et al. Social support and resilience in Black women affected by endometrial cancer. *Gynecol Oncol*. 2022; 226(1):145–149. PMID: 34481773.

Chapter 9

Berek J, Adams Hillard PJ. Initial assessment and communication. In: *Berek & Novak's Gynecology*, 16th ed. Alphen aan den Rijn, Netherlands: Wolters Kluwer, 2020:22–52.

Carusi D. The gynecologic history and pelvic examination. UpToDate. Wolters Kluwer. Accessed on March 17, 2025. https://www.uptodate.com/contents/the-gynecologic-history-and-pelvic-examination.

DynaMed. Ipswich (MA): EBSCO Information Services. 1995. Record No. T1647030685627, Gynecologic History and Pelvic Exam. Updated May 12, 2022. Accessed March 17, 2025. https://www.dynamed.com/topics/dmp~AN~T1647030685627.

Jain V, Munro M, Critchley HO. Contemporary evaluation of women and girls with abnormal uterine bleeding: FIGO Systems 1 and 2. *Int J Gynecol Obstet*. 2023;162(Suppl. 2):29–42. doi:10.1002/ijgo.14946.

Munro MG, Critchley HOD, Fraser IS, FIGO Menstrual Disorders Committee. The two FIGO systems for normal and abnormal uterine bleeding symptoms and classification of causes of abnormal uterine bleeding in the reproductive years: 2018 revisions. *Int J Gynaecol Obstet*. 2018;143:393–408. doi:10.1002/ijgo.12666.

Practice Bulletin No. 128: diagnosis of abnormal uterine bleeding in reproductive-aged women. *Obstet Gynecol*. 2012;120(1):197–206. doi:10.1097/AOG.0b013e318262e320.

Warner PE, Critchley HD, Lumsden MA, et al. Menorrhagia I: measured blood loss, clinical features, and outcome in women with heavy periods: a survey with follow-up data. *Am J Obstet Gynecol*. 2004;190:1216.

Finkelstein JS, Lee H, Karlamangla A, et al. Antimullerian hormone and impending menopause in late reproductive age: the study of women's health across the nation. *J Clin Endocrinol Metab*. 2020;105(4):e1862–e1871. doi:10.1210/clinem/dgz283.

Chapter 10

Tang B, Barnes K, Geers A, Livesey E, Colagiuri B. Choice and the placebo effect: a meta-analysis. *Ann Behav Med*. 2022;56(10):977–988. doi:10.1093/abm/kaab111.

Murray EJ. Editorial: demystifying the placebo effect. *Am J Epidemiol*. 2021;190(1):2–9. doi:10.1093/aje/kwaa162.

Kaptchuk TJ, Friedlander E, Kelley JM, et al. Placebos without deception: a randomized controlled trial in irritable bowel syndrome. *PLOS One*. 2010;5(12):e15591. Published December 22, 2010. doi:10.1371/journal.pone.0015591.

Fu S, Ke H, Yuan H, Xu H, Chen W, Zhao L. Dual role of pregnancy in breast cancer risk. *Gen Comp Endocrinol.* 2024;352:114501. doi: 10.1016/j.ygcen.2024.114501.

Gunter J. Yes, there's a new paper on hormonal contraception and breast cancer. *The Vajenda*. March 29, 2023. Accessed May 16, 2025. https://vajenda.substack.com/p/yes-theres-a-new-paper-on-hormonal.

Appendix B

Kaunitz, A. Abnormal uterine bleeding in nonpregnant reproductive-age patients: terminology, evaluation, and approach to diagnosis. UpToDate. Wolters Kluwer. Accessed April 10, 2025. https://www.uptodate.com/contents/abnormal-uterine-bleeding-in-nonpregnant-reproductive-age-patients-terminology-evaluation-and-approach-to-diagnosis.

Solone M, Adams Hillard PJ. Adult gynecology: reproductive years. In: *Berek & Novak's Gynecology*, 16th ed. Alphen aan den Rijn, Netherlands: Wolters Kluwer, 2020:316–355.

Index

Page numbers in *italics* refer to illustrations and tables

abdomen, 46
abdominal pain, 137, 152
abdominal palpation, 212
abdominal scan, 220
ablation, 135
ableism, 196
abnormal bleeding, 9–10, 216–22, *216–17*. *See also* heavy menstrual bleeding
  after age 60, 164–65
  defined, 63
  family history and, 254
  fibroids and, 137
  hysterectomies and, 64–65
  mistaken as vaginal or vulvar, *253*
  PALM-COEIN algorithm and, 218–20, 234
  postmenopausal, 164–65, 167–71, 176, 179, 235
  potential causes, *251–53*
  seeking help for, 224–25
  tests and, 220–25
  tracking symptoms, 217
abortion, 127, 143–44, 206
abuse, 34, 54, 160–61, 210
academic medical centers, 115
Accused, The (film), 20n
acid reflux, 146
acupuncture, 113
add-back therapy, 142
adenomyosis, 109, 219–20, 229, 255
adolescent gynecologists, 214
adrenal glands, 48
adrenal tumor, 171
adult diapers, 63, 138
AFAB (assigned female at birth), 4
agranulocytosis, 135n
Airhihenbuwa, Dr. Collins, 165
air pollution, 131
alcohol, 129
Alson, Julianna, 183
alternative medicine, 231–32
American College of Obstetricians and Gynecologists (ACOG), 167, 170n

American Journal of Obstetrics & Gynecology, 93
American Medical Association, 25
American Medical Society, 24
anal sphincter, 214
anarcha, 24–25
anatomy, 44–47
ancestral knowledge, 41
androgen, 74–75, 255
anemia, 5–6, 9, 64, 69–71, 85, 101, 137, 148, 166, 222
anesthesia, 25, 221
Angelou, Maya, 177, 193–94
anger squelching, 12, 131, 141, 255
anti-cancer diet, 226
anti-DEI rhetoric, 28
anti-inflammatory treatments, 108, 113
anti-Müllerian hormone (AMH), 222–23
anti-nausea medications, 33
antioxidants, 113
anti-progestins, 143
anus, 44, 47, 212
apoptosis, 107
appendix, 86
appraisal interval, 65n
aromatase enzyme, 126, 143, 255–56
aromatase inhibitors (AIs), 106, 143, 256
Asians and Pacific Islanders, 8, 158n
aspirin, 260
asymptomatic problems, 211
atrial fibrillation, 162
atrophy, 256
autoimmune conditions, 98n

Baby God (documentary), 211n
Baily, Moya, 201n
Baird, Dr. Donna, 148
Baralgin pills, 134–36
Bartholin's gland cysts, 213
Betsey, 24–25
Biden, Joseph, 38
bimanual exam, 213
biopsy, 166–67, 169–70, 179–80, 209, 220–21
biopsy pipette, 180, 220
birth control, 35, 49, 71–73, 99, 182, 207, 230
  combination, 77
  hormonal, 74, 127–28, 229, 230, 265
  low-dose progestin, 72–73
  pills, 127–28, 207
birth trauma, 24–25
Black Lives Matter, 146
Black maternal mortality, 3
Black STEM mentorship, 146, 155
Black women. *See also* silence, suffering and; Womb Sisters
  adaptation to pain and fatigue, 68
  advocacy groups for, 182–84, 249–50
  advocating for our own gynecological health, 237–38
  assumptions about strength of, 30, 33–34, 112
  cardiac catheterization study and, 112
  childbirth mortality, 154
  conditions of, inadequately treated, 9–10
  enslavement and, 8, 23–25, 40, 112
  feeling body and womb and, 194–97
  love letter to, 239–41
  medical profession and, 5–8, 30–32, 38, 40, 94–95, 111–12, 118, 162–63
  vocabulary for healthcare providers for, 235–37
Black women, disparities vs. White women.
  endometrial cancer and, 158–59, 162–63, 166–68, 172
  endometriosis and, 92, 103

fibroids and, 125–26, 137
hysterectomies and, 110
infertility and, 93
menopausal symptoms and, 170
surgical menopause and, 55n
Black Women's Health Study (BWHS), 127–31, *130,* 140–41
bladder, 10, 24, 44, 46, *47,* 108, 109, 118, 137, 142
bleeding. *See* abnormal bleeding; breakthrough bleeding; heavy menstrual bleeding; menstruation
bloating, 137
blood clots, 65, 77, 84, 141, 146–47, 219
blood-clotting factor, 53, 219
blood tests, 102, 221–22
Blue Cross Blue Shield, 7
BMI, 128
bone loss, 142
bowel, 109
bowel excisions, 108
bowel lesions, 108
bowel movements, pain and, 103–4, 120
Bradford, Joy Harden, 34
Bradley, Linda, 180
brain, 50, 98–99
breakthrough bleeding, 73, 76, 233, 235
breast cancer, 38, 158–59, 182, 230, 232
breastfeeding, 49, 127
breathing problems, 145–48, 233
Breslaw, Elaine, 23
Brown Jackson, Ketanji, 177
Brown University, 99, 110, 119
bruising, 253
bulk symptoms, 235

calcium, 113, 129
cancer, 6–7, 33, 36–37, 54, 60, 112, 117, 133, 151–54, 157–58, 166–67, 171, 175–76, 211, 219, 226–28, 232. *See also* cervical cancer; endometrial cancer; fibroids, cancer and, *and other specific types*
Canty, Ellen, 177–79, 181–82
Canty, Shakiya, 177–78, 181–82
Canty, Tikiya, 177–79, 181–82
capillary, 256
carbohydrates, 75
carboplatin, 175
carcinoma, 256
carcinosarcoma, 171, 256
cardiac catheterization, 112
cardiac muscle, 68
cardiovascular research, 36
Carolina Hysterectomy Cohort, 60n
CBC (complete blood count), 221–22, 256
celiac disease, 98n
cellular aging, 34
Centers for Disease Control (CDC), 162
certified nurse midwives, 265
cervical biopsies, 209
cervical cancer, 7, 9, 38, 67, 112, 158, 208, 226–27
cervical polyps, 213
cervix, 44–45, *45,* 54, 93, 211, 213, *252*
Chatman, Donald L., 93
chemotherapy, 173–75, 184n, 227
child abuse, 131
childbirth, 33, 80, 92, 127–28, 137–38, 154, 206, 254
childhood adversity, 172
China, 130
chlamydia, 208
Cierra Sister, 182
clear cell carcinoma, 171, 256
Cleveland Clinic, 180
clinical trials, 136, 179, 230
coagulopathy, 219, 223, 230

cognitive behavioral therapy, 113
Collins, Ms. Barbara, 159–64, 168–71, 173, 174, 176, 181
colon, 44, *47*, 104
colon cancer, 158, 257
colposcopy, 209
Columbia University, 28–29
Combahee River Collective, 165n
complex family planning, 264–65
condoms, 49
constipation, 137, 152
Cooper Owens, Deirdre, 23–24
copy number high endometrial cancer, 172n
Costco, 161
COVID-19, 114, 145, 162
COVID-19 vaccine, 38
COX-3 enzyme, 135
critical race theory, 165
C-section, 8, 24–25, 78
CT scan, 102, 147, 167
cycle syncing, 224, 256
cystectomy, 209
cysts, 213n

D&C (dilation and curettage), 256
dairy, 129n
Davis, Angela, 112
Deep South, 88
dehydration, 81
Delta Sigma Theta, 28, 188–89
dementia, 169
dental procedures, 254
Depends, 63
depression, 34, 105, 138
diabetes, 34, 36, 101
diagnosis and treatment, discussing options in, 234–35
diary or journal, 198, 207, 232–33
diclofenac, 141, 260
diet, 105–6, 114, 129, 140–41, 197, 219, 229
differential diagnosis, 234
digital tracking devices, 217n
dizziness, 81
DNA, 98, 172
dopamine agonists, 106
douching, 178
Duke University, 26–28, 192
dysplasia, 257

E2 (17beta-estradiol), 50n
ECANA (Endometrial Cancer Action Network for African Americans), 183–84, 190, 250n
ectopic pregnancy, 117
edema, 52
egg freezing, 149
eggs, 39–40, 46–48
elagolix, 106, 142
Elle Girl, 99
emotional freedom technique, 194
emotional vocabulary, 194
endocrine system, 68, 98
endocrinologist, 168
endometrial ablation, 78, 145
endometrial atrophy, 219
endometrial biopsy, 164, 179–81, 209, 220–21, 257
endometrial destabilization, 74–75
endometrial destruction, 78
endometrial fluid, 220
endometrial glands, 50
endometrial polyp, 257
endometrial stem cells, 53
endometrial thinning, 167
endometrial (uterine) cancer, 9, 10, 35, 43, 52n, 90, 157–84, 256
  attention to, 162–63
  biopsy and, 169–70, 173, 179–81
  Black vs. White disparities and, 5–7, 158–59, 166, 170–71
  Black women and aggressive, 167–68
  community outreach and, 182–84

deaths from, 177–78, 181
defined, 257
diagnosis of, 5–6, 60n, 158–59, 163–65, 166–72, 184n
doctors' lack of information about, 170
ECANA and, 183–84, 190
hysterectomy and, 24, 158
incidence rates, 158
mortality rates, 7, 158
pain and, 169–70
postmenopausal bleeding and, 167–69
research on, 25, 70, 163, 166
screening for, 163
stages of, 5–6, 181, 184n
surgery and, 173–74
treatment for, 174–76, 231
type 1 vs. type 2, 171
ultrasound and, 167, 170n
endometrioid carcinoma, 256
endometriosis, 5, 9–10, 35, 43, 91–120, 162, 209, 95–96, 99
asking gynecologist about, 120
Black vs. White disparities and, 92–94
Black women's rate of, 94–95
causes and process of, 96–97
cell migration and, 96–98, 107
cost of treatment, 101–2
defined, 257
delayed care and, 93–94
delaying childbearing and, 92–93
diagnosis of, 91–92, 99, 102–3, 119–20, 162–65, 233
extent of lesions, 108
failure to treat, 101
hormones and, 104–5, 107
impact of, 92
infertility and, 91
medical research and, 92–94, 162
"miracle cures," and, 229
misdiagnosed as PID, 93
myths about, 232
pain and, 90–92
pain and, after surgery, 114–20
pelvic exam and, 213
pregnancy and, 206
prevalence of, 98, 101–2
risk factors and, 94
screening for, 167
symptoms of, 102–3, 108, 167, 231
term coined, 92–93
treatment for, 92, 98, 101–20, 231
hormonal suppression, 104–5
second surgery, 117–19
supplements, 113–20
surgery, 107–12
ultrasound and, 103n
vitamins and, 12
endometriosis treatment and, side effects, 106–107
endometritis, 219, 257
endometrium
anatomy of, 45–47
basal layer, 52, 76, 78
breakthrough bleeding and, 73
defined, 257, 263
estrogen and, 50–51
fibroids and, 150
hysteroscopy and, 221
medications to decrease, 141
menstruation and, 48, 50, *51,* 52
removal of, 78–79
stabilization of, 74–78, 86
enslavement, 23, 30, 41, 61, 74
environmental pollution, 98, 129n, 172
enzymes, 52, 69
epidemiology, 60
epigallocatechin (EGCG), 140–41
epigenetics, 97–98, 139n
Essence Festival of Culture, 61
estradiol, 50n

estrogen, 223
 defined, 50n, 257–58
 endometrial cancer and, 171
 endometriosis and, 105–6, 109
 excess, 219
 fibroids and, 126–28, 131, 142, 143
 HMB and, 74–75
 menstrual cycle and, 50–51, *51,* 53
 soy and, 129
estrogen and progesterone medications, 53, 74, 76–77, 106, 114, 141–42
Eve, Dr. Paul, 24
excessive menstrual blood loss, 218
exercise, 75n, 114, 128–29, 141, 195–97, 199
extracellular matrix (ECM), 126

fallopian tubes, 40, *45,* 46, 91, 93, 223, *252,* 262
 cysts and, 220
 mass on, 117
family caregivers, 169, 173
family medicine, 265
fasting blood glucose levels, 223
fat cells, 74–75, 143, 171
fatigue, 68–69, 137
female pelvic medicine, 263–64
ferritin, 69, 70, 222, 258
fertility, 137–38, 150, 154, 221
fertility fraud, 211n
fetal development, 94
fetal kidney development, 122, 124
fiber, 197
fibroids (leiomyoma), 6, 9–10, 35, 43, 52n, 79, 117, 118, 121–56, 219
 anger suppression and, 12
 bleeding and, 167
 cancer and, 151–54
 defined, 79n, 126–27, 259
 degeneration of, 85–86, 89, 124
 diagnosis of, 135, 220
 diet and, 129
 early descriptions of, 125
 early menarche and, 127
 endometrium and, 46
 estrogen and, 126–27
 fairy-tale story of, 148–49
 gynecologic visit and, 209
 HMB and, 84–86, 90
 hysterectomy and, 90, 148–50
 inflammatory process and, 124
 intramural, 259
 IUDs and, 84n
 MIGS specialty and, 264
 misdiagnosis of cervical cancer as, 9
 myths about, 229–30, 232
 necrosis and, 124
 neglect of, 124, 154–56
 pelvic exam and, 211, 213
 pelvic MRI and, 261
 pregnancy and, 79–80, 123–24
 progesterone and, 127
 racial disparities and, 125
 risk factors and, 127–32, *130*
 size of, 122
 stem cells, 150
 submucosal, 221, 259
 subserosal, 259
 symptoms of, 124, 136–37, 155
 treatments for, 135, 139–56, 231
  medications, 141–44
  procedures, 144–49
  supplements and diet, 140–41
  surgery, 142, 149–56
First Nations, 175
first period. *See* menarche
fish, 129, 140
fish oil, 113
Fitzgerald, Dr. Jocelyn, 109n
Floyd, George, 201
follicle-stimulating hormone (FSH), 222
follicular phase, 51n

Ford, Dr. Chandra, 165
Foster, Jodie, 20n
frozen pelvis, 108n
fruits and vegetables, 129, 140

gender affirming specialists, 265
gender expansive people, 265
gender identity, 8
gene therapy, 175
genetics, 97–98, 167
genitals, shame and, 43
genital warts, 67n
Ghana, 27
Girl Scouts, 20
Giscombé, Cheryl Woods, 33–34
glycemic index, 129
GnRH agonists, 141–43
GnRH antagonist, 106, 142
gonorrhea, 208
Google, 72, 104
green tea, 140–41
Gunter, Dr. Jen, 230
gynecologic doctor
  access to, 188, 194–95, 198
  bedside manner, 248–49
  Black women's distrust of, 136
  finding, 111–12, 169, 247–50
  general, 263
  specialized, 249–50
  types of, 263–65
gynecologic health
  abnormal bleeding evaluation and, 216–20
  advocating for your own, 202–3, 237–38
  anatomy and, 44–47, *45*
  annual visit and, 203–10
  asking families about, 200
  healthcare system and, 7–8, 35–39
  importance of, 12–13, 182, 223–25
  importance of empathetic, 103, 114, 237–38
  listening to symptoms and, 224–25
  medical training and, 201
  mothers' advice on, 178–79
  miracle cure myths, 42, 229–30
  pelvic exam and, 210–15
  phases of life and, 47–56
  tests and lab studies, 220–25
gynecologic oncology, 7, 23, 40, 60, 108, 151, 169–70, 264
Gynecologic Research and Cancer Equity (GRACE) Center, 250n
gynecologic surgeons, 103
gynecologic visit
  assumptions about Black women and, 205
  bringing Womb Sister to, 204–5
  chaperone and, 205
  components of annual, 203–10
  first, 21–23, 66–68, 214
  guidelines for, 204
  importance of, 200
  history-taking interview, 204–10
  pelvic exam and, 66–68, 210–14
  review of systems, 210
  ways to make easier, 214–15
gynecologic vocabulary, 233–36
gynecology
  history of Black women and, 6, 23–26
  career in, 6–7, 26–32
  patient-centered care and, 224–25
  research and 37–98, 41, 103

hair loss, 34, 69–70
hair relaxers, 131
Hammond, Rev. Mary Elizabeth, 159
Hampton University, 134
Harris, Kamala, 177
Harvard University, 29, 60, 66
Hawk, Jereshia, 189–90
HBCUs (Historically Black College and University), 17, 134

head and neck cancers, 67n
healthcare, delay of, 65n
healthcare providers, 9, 198, 200, 235–36, 238
health equity, 37, 44
health insurance, 7, 29, 180
heart failure, 162
heavy menstrual bleeding (HMB), 9–10, 35, 43, 52n, 53, 59–90, 135. *See also* abnormal bleeding; menstruation
  anemia and, 64, 85
  Black women and, 166
  breaking through clothing, 49–50, 59
  causes of, 73
  defining, 63, 65, 218, *218,* 258
  diagnosis of, 63–66, 73n
  dizziness, dehydration, and pain and, 81–86
  excess estrogen and, 74–75
  exercise and, 75n
  experience of, 59–62
  failure to treat, 65–66
  fibroid degeneration and, 86–87
  fibroids and, 125, 135–36, 138–39, 143, 147
  insulin and, 75
  iron deficiency and, 71
  myths about, 232
  normalization of, 62
  onset of, 65n
  PALM-COEIN algorithm and, 218–20, 234
  prevalence of, 64
  progesterone IUD and, 80–81
  progestin and, 72
  as sign of broader disorder, 251–54
  suffering and silence about, 86–91
  sugar and, 12
  symptoms tracking, 217
  systemic conditions and, *253*
  treatment for, 73–78
    endometrial destruction, 78
    endometrial stabilization, 74–78
    hysterectomy, 78–79, 86–87
    medications, 141–43
HeLa cells, 38, 111n
hematocrit, 221, 258
hemoglobin, 69, 221, 223, 258
hemorrhage, 6
Hempstead, Bridgette, 182–83
heparin, 181
herpes, 208
high blood pressure (hypertension), 34, 162, 169, 196
histology, 171n, 258
HIV, 38, 208
holistic approach, 41–42, 128n, 131, 140, 182, 227, 232
hormonal implants, 74
hormonal suppression medication, 104
hormonal treatments, 108, 230–31
hormone replacement therapy, 171
hormones, 39, 48, 50, 54, 97, 105–7, 126, 258. *See also* estrogen; progesterone
  myths about, 230–31
hormone testing, 222–23
hot flashes, 55
human papillomavirus (HPV), vaccine, 67–68, 83, 208–9
Hutcherson, Dr. Hilda, 28
hydration, 124
hyperplasia, 219
hyper-sexualization, 35
hypothalamus, 48
hypoxia, 52, 53
hysterectomy, 6, 62, 64–65, 209, 258–59
  abdominal incision, 151
  Black vs. White disparities and, 10, 60, 88, 110

complete or simple, 259
complications, 151
endometrial cancer and, 24, 158, 168, 173–174
endometrial surgery and, 109–10
fibroids and, 90, 135, 148, 149–55
HMB and, 78–79, 86
laparoscopic or robotic, 151
loss of fertility and, 154
partial or subtotal, 259
sharing stories and, 191
uterine infection and, 90
vaginal, 151
hysteroscopic myomectomy, 150
hysteroscopy, 180, 221

iatrogenic condition, 219
ibuprofen, 21, 76, 82–83, 122, 136, 141, 146
Ifill, Gwen, 163, 177
imaging tests, 102–3
immune system, 53, 68, 98, 157
Immunotherapy, 175, 227
incontinence, 117, 138, 215–16
indomethacin, 260
infections, 89–90, 188, 208
infertility, 91–92, 122, 193–94, 209, 211, 223
infertility specialists, 211, 264
inflammation, 6, 52–54, 99, 107
inflammatory breakdown, 52n
inflammatory cascade of menstruation, 76–77
inflammatory pain, 113
inflammatory system, 98
informed consent, 136, 212
insulin, 75, 230
Internal Family Systems, 194
International Federation of Gynecology and Obstetrics, 219
intestines, 10
intimate partner violence, 54, 160–61, 210
iron, 68, 113
iron deficiency, 68–71, 137, 222
iron studies, 222
iron supplements, 70, 71, 135, 222
iron transfusions, 70, 85, 222
isoflavones, 129
IUD, 89, 230, 259. *See also* progesterone IUD
IVF treatments, 91, 122

Japanese people, 175
John Hopkins, 111n
Johns Hopkins University, 29
Johnson, Guy, 193–94
Johnson, Jasmine, 33
Jones, Tiffany Nicole, 177–78

Kaiser Permanente, 160
kidneys, 30, 36, 108
fetal, 124
Knowles-Carter, Beyoncé Giselle, 8

labia minora and majora, 212
Lacks, Henrietta, 38, 111–12
lactic ferments, 113
laparoscopic RF, 144
laparoscopy, 103–4, 108, 209, 264
Latinas, 8, 30, 33, 158n, 172
LEEPs, 209
leiomyoma, 125, 219, 259. *See also* fibroids
leiomyosarcoma, 151–53, 259
leuprolide acetate, 142
lichen sclerosis, 212–13
"lifestyle" diseases, 92n-93n
ligaments, *45,* 46
liver toxicity, 143
low birth weight, 94
low blood pressure, 64
Lucy, 24–25
lung cancer, 158
Lupron, 104, 106–7, 115
luteal phase, 51n, 52n

lycopene, 129
lymph nodes, 227
lymph system, 97

macrophages, 53
magnesium (mg), 113
magnetic resonance (MR) guided focused ultrasound, 145
malignancy, 219
mammograms, 162
Marsh, Erica, 128
massage therapy, 12
maternal fetal medicine, 123
maternal mortality, 154
McDowell, Ephraim, 24
Medicaid, 7, 29n
Medical Bondage (Owens), 23
Medical College of Georgia, 24
medical profession
  Black women's distrust of, 136
  harm to Black bodies and, 5, 227–28
medical research, 35–39, 43–44, 200–201
  doing your own, 232, 232n
  race and, 165–66, 201
Medicare, 7, 166
Meharry Hubbard Hospital, 17
Meigs, Dr. Charles, 24
Meigs, Dr. Joseph, 93–94, 100
melatonin, 113
memory, 197–98
menarche (first period), 48–49, 61–62, 94–96, 127, 133, 159–60, 191, 206, 259
  painful, 20, 120
MenoCheck picoAMH ELISA, 222n
menopausal hormone therapy, 230
menopause, 4, 54–56, 142, 163–64, 170, 179, 222–23, 259–60
  endometrium and, 219
  fibroids and, 148, 151
  pelvic exam and, 213
  spotting after, 10
  surgical, 55
menorrhagia, 63, 231, 260. *See also* heavy menstrual bleeding (HMB)
menstrual pain, 49–50, 59–60, 90, 134, 260. *See also* pain
  diet and, 231
  endometriosis and, 9, 91–94, 99–104, 108–9, 113–20
  fibroids and, 126
menstruation (menstrual cycle; period), 3–4. *See also* abnormal bleeding; heavy menstrual bleeding; menstrual pain
  abnormal, 10, 54
  adolescents and, 21
  Black women's as worst, 166
  defined, 50–51, 260
  endometriosis and, 97
  fibroids and, 89
  follicular phase, 260
  gynecologic visit and, 206
  heavy prolonged, 254
  hypoxia step, 52–53, 76n
  inflammation step, 52–54, 76n
  irregular, 53, 235
  lasting past age 60, 163–64
  length of period, 52n
  luteal phase of, 260
  menstrual phase, 51–53, *51*, 96–97
  mood disorders and, 216
  myths about, 228–29
  normal flow, *218*
  number of, 49, 97, 228–29
  PCPS and, 39
  perimenopause and menopause and, 54–55
  proliferative phase of, 260
  repair step, 52–54, 76n
  school and, 133–34
  secretory phase, *51,* 260

silencing about, 82–83
suppression of, 77–78, 115–16
tracking, 62, 72, 206
mental health support, 113. *See also* therapy
metamizole, 135n
Mexico, 130n
migraines, 34
migrated endometrium-like tissue, 105–6
MIGS (minimally invasive gynecologic surgeon), 104, 108, 114–15, 264
mindset, 195
mineral salts, 113
"miracle cures," 229–30
miscarriages, 127, 137, 178, 206
miscegenation laws, 92
misogynoir, 201
misogyny, 38, 201, 230
mitochondrial energy metabolism, 68
mood swings, 55
Moore, Adrienne, 184
morning-after pill, 143
Morrison, Toni, 177
motherhood, 37. *See also* childbirth; pregnancy
MRI, 102, 145, 261
mucinous carcinoma, 256
Murray, Dr., 168–69
muscle stem cell replication, fibroids and, 126
musculoskeletal system, 68
Myfembree, 142n
myocytes, 126, 139n
myomectomy, 135, 147, 150–51, 209, 260
myometrial stem cells, 126
myometrium, 126, 150
myths, 226–33

naproxen, 76, 141, 260
National Academy of Medicine, 38n
National Cancer Database, 6
National Cancer Institute (NCI), 36–37, 162
National Domestic Violence Hotline, 161n
National Heart, Lung, and Blood Institute, 36
National Institute for Health and Care Excellence, 63
National Institute of Child Health and Human Development (NICHD), 37, 38n
National Institute of Diabetes and Digestive and Kidney Diseases, 36
National Institute of Environmental Health Services (NIEHS), 37n
National Institute on Aging, 37
National Institutes of Health (NIH), 36–38, 163, 223
National Medical Association, 25
Native Americans, 8, 172, 175
nausea, 120
nervous system, 68, 98, 126
neuropathic pain, 113
neurotransmitter production, 68
New York Central Park, 25
New York Times, 79n
Nigerian immigrants, 17–19
nonbinary people, 265
nonhormonal medication, *252*
nonspecific symptoms, 102–3
norethindrone, 86, 142
North Carolina, 7, 33, 55n, 60n, 110, 118
symptom severity index, 88
Northwestern University, 201n
nosebleeds, 253
"not yet classified" condition, 220
NSAIDs, 76–77, 83, 113, 124, 141, 260
Nyong'o, Lupita, 40n

obesity, 128n, 182
OB-GYN residency, 5, 29, 60
obstetrical history, 206
off-label uses, 143
Olugbemi, Omotayo (grandmother), 17, 241
omega-3s, 113, 129n
oophorectomy, 24, 54–55, 109, 209, 261
Oriahnn, 142n
os, 45, *45*, 213
Our Father (documentary), 211n
ovarian cancer, 7, 39–40, 78n
ovarian cystectomy, 261
ovaries, 39, 40, 220, 223
  anatomy and function of, *45*, 46–48
  bleeding and, *252*
  cysts and, 209, 220, 254
  endometriosis and, 91, 108–9
  estrogen and, 74, 109
  hormones and, 50, 54
  hysterectomy and, 149
  menopause and, 54
  menstruation and, 48, 50, 53
  STIs and PID and, 93
  surgical removal of, 24, 54–55, 109
  tumors and, 171, 223
ovulation, 50, 51n, 53, 75, 197, 261
  ovarian cancer and, 78n
  suppression of, 49, 77–78
ovulatory dysfunction, 219, 222
OWN network, 177

P4 (pregn-4-ene-3,20-dione), 50n
paclitaxel, 175
pain. *See also* menstrual pain; pelvic pain; sex, painful
  biopsy and, 221
  Black vs. White women and, 5, 33, 68
  endometrial cancer and, 169
  endometriosis and, 92–93, 99–104, 108–9, 113–20
  fibroids and, 122–24, 126, 137
  physical activity and, 196
  pushing through, 30, 124
  ratings, 33, 87
pain medications, 33. *See also* NSAIDs; *and specific types*
  biopsy and, 221
PALM-COEIN algorithm, 218–20, 234
palpitations, 55
pancreas surgery, 121
panic attacks, 34
Pap smear, 22, 63–65, 111–112, 118, 162–65, 208–9, 211
paracervical block, 179–80, 221
pathologists, 171n, 174
PBS NewsHour (TV show), 177
pediatric health, 37
pelvic exam, 68n, 210–15
  chaperone and, 205
  need for regular, 210–12
  what to expect in, 212–15
pelvic floor disorders, 117, 215, 216, 264
pelvic floor physical therapists, 113
pelvic inflammatory disease (PID), 5, 208, 261
  endometriosis misdiagnosed as, 93, 100–101
pelvic pain, 5, 53, 85, 215–16
  endometriosis and, 102, 120
  after endometriosis surgery, 113
pelvic pain specialist, 215
pelvic pressure, 137–38
pelvic ultrasound, 220
pelvis, organs inside, 46
penis biopsy, 109n
penis lesion removal, 109n
perimenopause, 54–55, 170, 261
perineum, 212

period. *See* abnormal bleeding; menarche; heavy menstrual bleeding; menstrual pain; menstruation
peritoneum, 97, 103, 261
Pettway, Jessica, 9
pharmaceutical companies, 36, 231
"Phenomenal Woman" (Angelou), 177
Philadelphia medical museum, 24
phytoestrogens, 129
pituitary gland, 48
placebo effect, 229–30
plasmin, 77
platinum, 175
platelets, 222
pluripotent cells, 98n
Poland, 130
polio vaccine, 38
pollution, 37n
polycystic ovary syndrome (PCOS), 39, 209, 219, 230
polyps, 46, 167, 219, 221, 230
postpartum pelvic trauma, 264
pre-cancer, 219
preeclampsia, 8, 196
pregnancy, 34, 37–38, 49, 137, 160, 188, 196, 206, 230. *See also* birth control; infertility
  early rupture of membranes, 79–80, 83, 138
  endometriosis and, 92
  fear of, 181–82
  fibroids and, 79, 80, 122–24, 137–38, 154
  IVF treatments, 91
  morning-after pill, 143
  number of monthly cycles and, 229
  perimenopause and, 54
  prevention of, 35, 71–72
premenarche, 47–48
Prentice Ambulatory Care (PAC), 29–30
Prentice Women's Hospital, 5–6, 29–32
presidential elections of 2024, 38
Prevost, François-Marie, 24
Procedures, surgery vs., 144
progesterone, 143
  defined, 50n, 261
  endometriosis and, 106
  fibroids and, 127, 131, 139n, 142
  HMB and, 75–76
  menstruation and, 50–52
  testing for, 222–23
progesterone IUDs, 74, 76, 80, 83, 118, 141, 197
  expulsion pf, 84, 141
progesterone patch or implants, 76. *See also* estrogen and progesterone medications
progestins, 50n, 261
prolapse, 117, 214, 215
proliferative phase of endometrium, 50
prostaglandins, 52, 135n, 141, 262
proteins, 69, 98
psoriasis, 98n
puberty, 48, 96
public health, 182–83
Public Health Critical Race praxis, 165
pulmonary embolus, 8

race. *See also* Black women, disparities vs. White women
  funding of scientists and, 37
  hysterectomy and, 60
race-stratified data, 7
racial and gender stereotypes, 34
racism, 4–5, 11–12, 28, 33, 100, 130, 132, 134, 195, 199–200, 201, 228
radiation, 173, 174, 184n, 227
radiofrequency ablation (RF), 144–45
rape, 20, 40n, 61

Read, The (podcast), 233
rectovaginal exam, 213–14
red blood cells, 68, 69, 70, 221
relugolix, 106, 142
reproductive endocrinology, 264
respiratory polyps, 67n
Reynolds, Mary, 23–24
rheumatoid arthritis (RA), 98n, 101
Rios-Doria, Dr. Eric, 172
Risques, Dr. Rosana, 172
Rivers, Louis, III, 68, 71–72, 79–80
RNA, 98
Roberson, Dr. Mya, 94–95, 99–101, 103–5, 107–8, 110–12, 114–20, 233
Robinson, Dr. Whitney Ragan, 60–63, 66–67, 71–72, 79–89, 110, 233
robotic surgery, 173, 264
Rose, Dr., 132–36, 138–39, 145–50, 154–56, 233

Sage, Liz, 183
salicin, 260
saline-infusion sonohystogram (SIS), 221
salpingectomy, 209, 262
salpingo-oophorectomy, 262
  bilateral (BSO), 262
  unilateral (USO), 262
Sampson, Dr. John, 92–93, 100
Seattle Times, 161
selective estrogen receptor modulators (SERMs), 106
selective progesterone receptor modulators (SPRMs), 106, 143
self-care, 34
  prioritizing, 188
selenium (Se), 113
sensory nerve cells, 98–99
serosa of uterus, 150
serous carcinoma, 169–71, 256
Set Boundaries, Find Peace (Tawwab), 34
sex, painful
  endometriosis and, 103, 105, 113–14, 117, 120
  fibroids and, 125, 137
sex education, 20, 132–33
sexism, 11, 195
sexual history, gynecologic visit and, 206–7
sexually transmitted infections (STIs), 5, 93, 100–101, 132, 211
sexual orientation, 207
sexual violence, 54
silence, suffering and, 3, 5, 9, 17, 19, 21, 35, 40–41, 71, 81–82, 90, 94, 133, 155, 177–78
  breaking from, 183, 187, 189, 199–201, 207n, 224
  normalization of suffering and, 63–64
Simply Soulful Café, 161, 169
Sims, Dr. J. Marion, 24–25
skin cells, 143
skin conditions, 212–13
sleep, 34, 98, 114, 197
Smith, Dr., 72, 73
social media, 9, 179, 231–32
Society of Gynecologic Oncology, 174–75, 183
somatic mutations, 98, 262
somatic therapy, 194
sonohystogram, 221
soy, 129
speculum, 45, 213–15
spirituality, 228
spotting, post-menopause, 10
stem cells, 126, 139n, 150, 262
Stevens-Johnson syndrome, *253*
"Still I Rise" (Angelou), 177
strength, 34–35
stress, 34, 53, 98, 131, 172, 193
  endometriosis and, 92–93, 114
  fibroids and, 131, 141
  weathering and, 263

Stroger Hospital of Cook County, 6, 64
stroma, 256
Study of Women's Health Across the Nation (SWAN), 222
Stuebe, Dr. Alison, 33
sugar, dietary, 12, 75, 129, 230
suicidal ideation, 105
Superwoman Schema (Giscombé), 33–34
supplements, 113, 140–41, 229
surgery. *See also* hysterectomy; *and other specific types*
  care team and, 173–74
  endometrial cancer and, 173–74
  endometriosis and, 102–4, 107–12
  previous, gynecologic visit and, 209
  procedures vs., 144
  unexpected bleeding and, 254
surrogacy, 154
swim class, periods and, 134
Swisher, Dr. Elizabeth, 172
symptoms, 188, 198–99, 207–8, 232–36
  diary of, 198, 207, 232–33
  gynecologic visit and, 207–9
  vocabulary and, 233–35

TAH/BSO, 262
Taverna-Miller, Dr. Karen, 104–5, 110, 112, 115–16
Tawwab, Nedra Glover, 34
teen pregnancy, 132, 155
Teen Vogue, 99
telehealth, 146
TheHotline.org, 161n
therapy, 192–94, 199, 200
Therapy for Black Girls, 34
thyroid, 48, 101, 162, 168
thyroid studies (TSH), 223
TLH/BSO, 262
Tomashek, Holly, 174
Towolawi, Dr. Margaret, 70
toxins, 37n, 131
TP53 tumor suppressor gene mutations, 171, 172
tranexamic acid, 77, 86, 141
transcervical procedures, 144
trans people, 4, 265
transvaginal ultrasound (TVUS), 122, 167, 170n, 220, 262
trauma, *252*
Tumor Board, 124–25
tumor vaccines, 175
Turkey, 130
12 Years a Slave (film), 40n

ulipristal acetate, 143
ultrasound
  biopsy and, 167
  cysts, 213n
  endometrial cancer and, 167–68
  endometriosis and, 102, 103n, 117
  fibroids and, 123–24, 147
University of California, San Francisco, 29
University of Michigan, 68
University of North Carolina, 7, 60
University of Pennsylvania, 29
University of Virginia, 32–33
UpToDate, 232
ureter, 108, 262–63
urethra, 44, *47,* 212
urethral polyps, 213
urination, 120. *See also* incontinence
  frequent, 117, 118, 137–38
  leakage and, 24–25
  painful, 120
urogenital fistulas, 24–25
urogynecologist, 117, 214–15, 263–64
US Congress, 38
US Public Health Service Untreated Syphilis Study at Tuskegee, 38
uterine artery embolization (UAE), 135, 144

uterine cancer. *See* endometrial cancer
uterine-sparing treatments, 110, 263
uterus, 6, 39. *See also* endometriosis; endometrium; hysterectomy; *and specific parts*
- bleeding and, *252*
- contraction and relaxation of, 126
- defined, 45–46, *45, 47,* 48, 263
- endometriosis and, 91, 96–98
- endometriosis surgery and, 109–10
- fallopian tubes and, 40
- fibroids and, 125–26, 137
- infections and, 86–90
- layers of, *51*
- muscle wall, 52
- myometrium and, 126, 263
- pelvic exam and, 213
- perimenopause and, 54
- STDs and, 93
- subserosa, 263
- urogenital fistulas and, 24

vagina, 40, 44, *45, 47,* 48, 223
- bleeding and, 5, *251*
- cancers of, 67n
- pelvic exam and, 213–14
- precancerous lesions and, 211
- STDs and, 93
- urogenital fistulas and, 24

vaginal biopsy, 109n
vaginal cancer, 7
vaginal dryness, 55
vaginal lesion removal, 109n
vaginal ring, 76
vaginal suppositories, 178
vaginal walls, 54
Vanderbilt University, 116
vascular system, 98
vegan diet, 129n
VEGF inhibitors, 175
vitamin A, 113
vitamin B6, 113, 140
vitamin C, 113
vitamin D, 113, 129, 130–31, 140–41
vitamin E, 113, 227
vitamins, 12
vomiting, 120
vulnerability, 34, 123–25
vulva, 40, 212, 223
- bleeding, *251*

vulvar cancer, 7, 67n, 213
vulvar pain, 85

Walters, Barbara, 163
weathering, 263
WebMD, 232
weight gain, 34
wellness influencers, 12, 41–42
West, Crissle, 233
West Africans, 23
West Indies, 132
Whipple surgery, 121
white blood cell count, 89–90
White doctors, 23–24, 31–32, 67–68, 135, 164
White women, 35, 55n, 110, 112. *See also* Black women, disparities vs. White women
Williams, Serena, 8
Willis, Marjorie "Margie," 182–83
Winfrey, Orpah, 177
Womb. *See also* uterus
- Black women and cancers of, 35
- biomedical research and, 37
- cyclical clock and, 50
- everyday nonpregnant, 201
- feeling, 194–97
- healing and, 199–201
- love of, 39–42
- impact of problems of, on society, 39
- prioritizing health of, 188, 191
- reason for focus on, 40

Womb Sisters, 4, 9, 15, 188–91, 201
- annual gynecologic visit, 204–5

womb stories, 182, 189–92
Womb Strength, 39, 71
Womb Suffering
  Black women and, 35
  breaking cycle of, 4, 192
  challenging normalized, 11
  giving Black women tools to unlearn, 12–13
  gynecologic treatments to ease, 54
  normalization of, 4, 9, 13
  self-sufficiency and, 35
  stigma of treatments for, 35
Women, Race & Class (Davis), 112
women of color, 195n
women's health, underfunding of, 37–38, 41, 44, 103, 109, 231
women's healthcare, scarcity of, 164–65
women's health nurse practitioners, 265
World Health Organization, 258
wounds, minor, 253
Wright, Dr. Maya, 55n

yeast infections, 178n, 208
yoga, 113, 196
Yoruba tribe, 18

zinc (Zn), 113

ABOUT THE AUTHOR

DR. KEMI DOLL is a physician, surgeon, advocate, career coach, and a double board-certified gynecologic oncologist and uterine cancer scientist. She is a professor on faculty in the Department of Obstetrics and Gynecology at the University of Washington School of Medicine and an adjunct professor in the Department of Health Systems and Population Health at the University of Washington School of Public Health, where she directs the Gynecologic Research and Cancer Equity (GRACE) Center. She lives in Seattle, Washington, with her family.

ABOUT THE TYPE

This book was set in Garamond, a typeface originally designed by the Parisian type cutter Claude Garamond (c. 1500–61). This version of Garamond was modeled on a 1592 specimen sheet from the Egenolff-Berner foundry, which was produced from types assumed to have been brought to Frankfurt by the punch cutter Jacques Sabon (c. 1520–80).

Claude Garamond's distinguished romans and italics first appeared in *Opera Ciceronis* in 1543–44. The Garamond types are clear, open, and elegant.